Coping with Dementia

Laura Town and Karen Hoffman

Omega Press

Zionsville, IN 46077

ISBN-13: 978-0-9969832-9-7

Production Credits:
Authors: Laura Town and Karen Hoffman
Publisher: Omega Press
Contributor: Sean Dixon
Photos: All images used under license from Shutterstock.com

Social media connections:
Laura Town
Twitter: @laurawtown
LinkedIn: https://www.linkedin.com/in/lauratown
Facebook: https://www.facebook.com/omegabookpublishers/

Karen Hoffman
LinkedIn: https://www.linkedin.com/in/karen-hoffman-91502b62/

CONTENTS

COPING WITH DEMENTIA

People, whether they be friends or strangers, will be sympathetic when you tell them that a loved one has dementia. Not knowing how to respond, people will try to find something positive to say about your tragedy—and dementia is tragic. The one comment that bothered me (Laura) the most, although the intention behind it was good, was that at least my father "doesn't know what's happening to him." This is completely false. My dad, in the early and even in the mid stages, knew what was happening. Yes, he couldn't articulate it all the time. Yes, he could not go into detail about the functions of the brain or give a scientific explanation of what was happening. But he knew that he could no longer complete simple tasks. He cried when he could no longer drive. He was enraged when he could not remember the names of his relatives. And he sank into a deep depression when he had to start wearing adult diapers. Even in the late stages when dad was living in a locked dementia unit and before he became nonverbal, my father pointed to adults rocking baby dolls and said to me that he wished he wasn't one of "those people."

Dad's doctor told me that if you've seen one case of Alzheimer's disease, it just means that you've seen one case of Alzheimer's disease, meaning that all cases are different. Perhaps some people slide straight from complete cognition to the late stages of Alzheimer's disease and truly do not have any frustration while being in the throes of the disease, but I have never heard of this.

So people with dementia do know, on a fundamental level, what is happening. That doesn't mean that they know it every day, or even every hour, or become obsessed with their declining health. Dad still had happy moments. He still enjoyed taking walks, listening to music, seeing his grandsons, and eating cupcakes. As long as he was able, I still took him out to restaurants for lunch and dinner or brought him to my house. And although he wasn't particularly religious, he enjoyed visits with the ministers and volunteers who came and read the Bible to him. The challenge is to find what your loved one enjoys and then try to incorporate the enjoyment of it into as many moments of their life as you are able. If you are the one suffering from dementia, then think about what gives you pleasure and find a way to do those things as often as you are able.

When your loved one is diagnosed with Alzheimer's disease or another type of dementia, the emotional effect on the whole family is tremendous. As much as possible, the person with dementia has to come to terms with living with a terminal degenerative disease. They must reckon with a failing memory as well as an increasing reliance on others while also dealing with a society that may feel they have lost their value. Once they enter middle- and later-stage dementia, the disease will begin to affect emotional responses as well as the ability to communicate.

Caregivers, family, and friends of the person with dementia must also process powerful emotions about the news. If your parent, spouse, or other loved one is diagnosed with dementia, you might experience grief over your loved one's loss of memory as well as confusion and stress over practical medical, legal, and financial issues. Your family will likely face some major challenges as you collectively adapt to meet the new needs of the person with dementia. Most significantly, the day-to-day stress of caregiving can take a profound toll on your physical and mental well-being. Being a caregiver affects all parts of your life—personal, professional, and financial—and you may feel that you don't have more than a few minutes to yourself each day. This daily stress can continue for years—sometimes a decade or longer—with serious health implications for you and your family. Studies have found that caregivers' own health problems can be caused or exacerbated by the constant stress of providing care. Studies have also shown that stressed caregivers effectively age faster than people without chronic caregiving responsibilities. According to an American Association of Retired Persons (AARP) report from 2015, 34.2 million Americans provided unpaid care to an adult age 50 or older in the prior 12 months. According to the same report, caregivers spend an average of 24.4 hours a week providing care, with nearly a quarter spending 41 hours or more on care each week, and those caring for a spouse or partner spending 44.6 hours a week. That's an enormous time investment that leaves significantly less time for paid employment and leisure activities. It's easy to see from this how easily caregiving can become all-consuming for the people who provide it.

This book examines the emotional fallout of dementia, and specifically how people with the disease, their caregivers, and their non-caregiver family and friends can cope with that fallout. You'll read about the stages of the disease and how to cope with the common changes at each step. You'll also read about problems that often accompany a terminal chronic illness such as Alzheimer's disease—depression, anxiety, anger, guilt, sleep disturbances, and suicide risk—and how to respond healthily to each of these problems. You'll also get tips and advice for how to support others over the course of dementia: the loved one with the disease, other caregivers, and other family and friends. Although there are different types of dementia including Alzheimer's disease, our checklists should be applicable regardless of the specific diagnosis, and so "dementia" is the term used throughout this book for Alzheimer's disease and other types.

Emotional Considerations for the Individual with Dementia

Dementia destroys the cognitive function of the individual with the disease. Its effects are catastrophic. The reality is that if you have dementia, you will not only lose the ability to think and remember clearly. You will experience extreme behavioral and emotional changes as the disease progresses, will no longer recognize family members or close friends, and may even develop irrational fears and paranoias. Everyone experiences a loss of function and independence as they age. This is often an emotional struggle. But for people with dementia, these normal changes are compounded in every way and are accompanied by other fundamental changes in how they think, speak, and act.

If you have been diagnosed with dementia, all of this will be painful and overwhelming to confront. This is why the first thing you need to do when you are diagnosed, the only thing you need to do, is allow yourself to experience your emotions. This will be different for every person, but this process is very likely to be similar to the stages of grief as defined by the psychiatrist Elisabeth Kübler-Ross: denial, anger, bargaining, depression, and, finally, acceptance. Give yourself the time and permission to experience and move through these emotions. If you need to feel angry, feel angry. If you need to feel depressed, feel depressed. Try not to lash out at others, but experience all the emotions it's natural to feel at this time. Try to talk to other people about how you feel and try not to isolate yourself, but at the same time, do what you need to do. Don't be ashamed of anything you feel right now. Your emotions are telling you what you need. Listen. There will be a time for understanding and for making important decisions, but that time is not when you are first diagnosed. This time is for you to figure out a way to confront this disease that seems most natural to you.

Once you have experienced the emotions you need to experience, then it is time to seek help to get some of the legal and financial documents you need in place. You won't want to think about this, but it is important to do now while you can still think clearly and make these important decisions for yourself. You can get help with this from your loved ones and learn the basics steps by reading *Long-Term Care Insurance, Power of Attorney, Wealth Management, and Other First Steps*. These first steps come with their own emotional struggles, and it's okay to embrace and experience those emotions, too. You're not alone in this, and whenever you need it, ask for help along the way.

The next two sections examine how to begin understanding the progression of dementia and coping with the diagnosis from the perspective of the individual with the disease. Then the following section turns to the caregiver to suggest ways that caregivers can help with that coping.

How Dementia Progresses

One thing that may help you if you have been diagnosed with dementia is to learn what the disease is and what it does. Probably the best way to approach understanding dementia is to learn what you should expect as the disease progresses. Although the effects of dementia and how it progresses are different for everyone who has it, generally people with dementia experience a gradual worsening of symptoms over time. In the early stages, memory loss and reduction of ability to function are minor and very gradual, but in the later phases, people with dementia lose the ability to participate in give-and-take conversation and react to stimuli. If you have dementia, activities you used to do easily, such as balancing a checkbook or keeping track of your keys, will become gradually more difficult. The checklist below focuses on the early changes to expect.

Checklist: Early changes to expect with dementia

- ☐ Disruptive memory loss, such as forgetting information you learned recently and important dates and events. You may ask for the same information again and again, but you may not remember that you've already asked for it.

- ☐ Difficulty solving problems, such planning an event and keeping track of bills. Working with numbers or following processes with many steps may become especially difficult.

- ☐ Being confused about time and place. You may have trouble remembering what day it is, why you are where you are and what you were doing, or what is happening right now.

- ☐ Misplacing things, such as not finding car keys where you expect them to be.

- ☐ Difficulty performing familiar work or personal tasks. This may make it challenging or impossible to continue working if you are not retired.

- ☐ Problems with self-expression, such as difficulty organizing thoughts or finding the right words to say what you mean. This may make it difficult for you to follow conversations or to take an active part in them.

- ☐ Impaired judgment that compromises decision making. This may be difficult for you to be aware of, but if you think you've paid for a good or service you haven't received, you notice charges that don't look right to you in your credit card statements, or you receive strange bills, ask for help from your caregivers in understanding what concerns you.

- ☐ Changes in mood and personality, such as depression, anxiety, or sudden and unpredictable irritability and anger. You may become socially withdrawn, even if you are normally very social, and you may lose motivation to complete tasks, especially challenging ones.

How to Cope if You Have Been Diagnosed with Dementia

If you feel embarrassed by your symptoms and are afraid to talk to others or ask for help, you are not alone. Many people with dementia experience this. However, trying to cover up the symptoms can be very stressful, and eventually it's impossible to cover up the signs. Instead, you should try to integrate changes from the disease into daily life while remaining as active and engaged as possible. If you have been diagnosed, remember to be flexible, fine-tune your approach from day to day, and ask for help. Although some people stigmatize the need to depend on others as weak and parasitic, it is wrong to view relationships this way, especially your relationships with close family and friends. People help one another not just out of a sense of obligation but also to find meaning and purpose in their own lives. If you let other people help you, you can better cope with the disease, and you may also help them cope better with it as well by giving them a way to deal with it. Remember: You and the ones who love and care for you are all in this together.

Checklist: How to cope with a diagnosis of dementia

- ☐ Research dementia and discuss your feelings and findings with loved ones.

- ☐ Involve family and friends in your efforts to learn all you can about dementia.

- ☐ Ask all medical providers to explain medical terms and instructions that you find confusing or do not remember. Encourage a close family member or friend to assist you in these efforts, helping you take note of anything important for you to know about your diagnosis.

- ☐ Find out what support services are available in your community. Local organizations may offer everything from transportation help to peer counseling.

□ Decide who your primary caregivers should be and, with their help, begin creating and organizing a daily routine for yourself.

□ If you feel overwhelmed with depression, anxiety, and stress following your diagnosis, don't hesitate to seek out a mental health provider. Meeting with a mental health professional early in the course of the disease can help you cope better as the condition worsens. For information on finding a mental health provider, see the Resources at the end of this book.

Ways That Caregivers Can Help an Individual Cope with Dementia

To handle the problems of early-stage dementia—such as losing keys, forgetting phone numbers, and having more difficulty managing money—and their associated frustration, the individual with dementia will need help from others. This is inevitable. Caregivers can develop strategies to help the individual with dementia mitigate confusion and frustration. Because loss of memory and general cognitive function are a part of dementia from its earliest stage, the following checklists are aimed at caregivers assisting the individual.

Checklist: Developing a coping strategy

□ Take note of changes in the abilities of the individual with dementia. Look for evidence of erratic purchases online or frequently losing track of household tasks. Make a list of the tasks that you observe have become more difficult for the person with dementia.

□ To determine which tasks to address first, determine their relative importance. For example, between trouble writing checks and losing house keys, it may be most important to address the key problem first because this is likely to be a daily need.

□ Priorities such as writing checks may be something you can automate. Any bill payment that can be automated to take place at a specific time each month without the individual's intervention should be. For any other bill, keep track of when the bill is due and then assist the individual with making payments at the appropriate times. You might use a calendar to note important things, drawing a big X over completed days so the person can more easily tell what day it is and what tasks they need to do that day.

☐ For items that the individual frequently misplaces, such as keys, take care to watch where the individual places them. If the individual puts these items down in random places, put them in a consistent place. This can help you keep better track of these items, and it may help the individual as well. Watch the individual several times because it may clue you in to patterns or hiding places that you otherwise wouldn't have thought about. Then once you have noticed a pattern (if there is one), make a spot where that item goes close to where the person habitually puts them.

☐ In addition to placing keys and similar items in designated places, consider using signs such as "Leave keys here" to help the individual remember. Use a picture or a picture and words if you think that would be easier. Anything that helps is worth trying, but respect the individual's preferences.

Checklist: Helping the individual with early-stage dementia maintain a good attitude

☐ Help the individual focus on the moment and set realistically achievable goals.

☐ Try not to argue with the individual even when they repeatedly say things that make no sense or appear to see things that are not there. For example, my (Laura's) father kept "seeing" and "talking" to his dead mother. I didn't' tell him that she's dead, because it didn't really matter at that time and he found comfort in the conversations. If the individual becomes agitated, try to gently redirect the individual toward something else.

☐ Create reminders, patterns of behavior, and social networks that help the individual navigate through each day successfully. Involve the individual's family and friends in these activities when you can.

- Create a routine for the individual. Each day, make a plan to ensure that the individual accomplishes what they need to that day. Keep these plans small and realistic, and be ready to step in whenever necessary to provide guidance. Scheduling can reduce confusion and limit the amount of time you need to spend planning. This can also orient you toward completing the most necessary tasks first.

- Take on tasks individually. Move on if the individual can't complete a task in the moment. If a task becomes too difficult and frustrating for the individual, have the individual take a break, but remember to return to the task again later and provide whatever help the individual needs to complete it. The individual with dementia will likely not remember the task or where they left off with it, so you will need to remind them.

- You and the individual will have multiple chances to solve most problems. If one strategy for locating keys or remembering phone numbers is not working, you can always develop another technique to achieve your goal. Talk to other caregivers about which strategies they are using that might help.

- Identify the events or thoughts that cause the individual stress, such as becoming distressed when others do not fully explain their intentions. Being aware of these stress triggers can help you manage them. If anything that makes the individual unhappy or stressed can simply be removed, then do so.

- Discover sources of strength for the individual and use them. When prayer, a pet, spending time with family or friends, listening to music, or a hobby fills the individual with joy, encourage the individual to devote time to that activity to get them through difficult patches.

- Music can be an amazing tool for caregivers. It can boost brain activity by evoking emotions that bring back memories; inspire emotional and physical closeness; reduce anxiety, depression, and agitation; and elevate the mood of the individual with dementia while lowering stress. Musical aptitude and appreciation are among the last abilities that remain for individuals with dementia. When using music, be careful to set the mood, choose music you know the individual likes, and encourage movement while watching your loved one's reaction and avoiding overstimulation. Sing along and have fun with it.

Managing the individual's physical and emotional health depends on taking a holistic approach; for example, managing physical health can improve emotional health, and vice versa.

Checklist: Managing the health of an individual with dementia

☐ Give care in a way that focuses on potential and strength rather than the individual's lost abilities. Ensure that they feel useful by building on their abilities. Provide opportunities for your loved one to make choices. For example, if your loved one used to love cooking, but you feel they can no longer use the stove or oven or knives safely, then think of kitchen tasks your loved one can do such as washing vegetables or mixing ingredients. Some tasks your loved one may not be able to do on their own but could do with supervision, such as using the microwave, measuring ingredients, or reading a recipe.

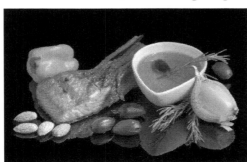

Instead of asking questions to test their ability (do you know where the butter is?) that they may not be able to answer, get out ingredients for them or hand them the right ingredients to support them in tasks they can still do. The same process can be used for cleaning, laundry, financial tasks, etc.

Credit: Sergey Yechikov

☐ Avoid imposing expectations on the individual that are based on their previous values or abilities.

☐ Establish a relationship with a physician the individual trusts and see them regularly.

☐ Create a balanced diet plan and a regular exercise routine. A balanced diet has not necessarily been shown to alleviate the symptoms of dementia, but heart-healthy eating patterns such as the Mediterranean diet have been shown to contribute to overall well-being and longevity. (See *Nutrition for Brain Health: Fighting Dementia* for more information on how to eat a brain-healthy balanced diet.)

☐ The diet plan should also improve physical well-being. Food rich in essential minerals and vitamins tend to increase alertness and create hormones that can inspire greater emotional health.

☐ Encourage the individual to exercise regularly. Multiple scientific studies have demonstrated the ability of physical activity to slow a decline in cognition and memory. Mild-to-moderate exercise also reduces the symptoms of depression, anxiety, stress, and even the risk of falls.

☐ Build a network of people who understand the individual's needs and can help keep track of their emotional and physical health. Try to maximize the individual's contact with people who bring the individual joy. Make contact with others face to face whenever possible.

☐ Encourage the individual to take breaks when they are tired. Help them get back on track with uncompleted tasks later.

☐ Ensure the individual limits drinking alcohol to only a small amount.

☐ Check with a doctor before the individual changes medications or dosages. Help the individual maintain compliance with their medication schedule. Be alert to any changes in their drug regimen to ensure continued compliance.

☐ If they are up to it, help the individual engage in activities they enjoy to increase brain activity and connect with others socially. For example, they may join a book club, volunteer, play an instrument, or learn new hobbies. Mental stimulation has not been conclusively shown to slow the progression of dementia, but engaging in meaningful activities does contribute to a feeling of well-being for many people, and learning new skills may improve the ability to think as well.

☐ Encourage the individual to talk to someone they trust about their emotions. Help them to express themselves the best they can. The better you understand how the individual feels, the more likely you will be able to respond in appropriate ways.

☐ Ensure the individual does not ignore their spiritual life, which can help provide context for their feelings and give them a sense of a relationship with something larger than themselves. Encourage whatever spiritual practice gives them a sense of peace, whether that's going outdoors, meditating, singing hymns, or praying.

☐ Encourage the individual to seek and accept help from loved ones and caregivers, and be sure to do the same yourself. Someone else may be able to assist you in helping the individual to reach a physical or emotional health goal.

☐ Have the individual talk to a mental health professional if they find that the stress or confusion of the diagnosis is overwhelming on a regular basis. Talk to the mental health professional yourself to develop strategies to help the individual regain a feeling of control.

☐ Use any support services that medical providers and local community resources provide, especially if they are free.

Eventually, the individual with dementia will be less capable of communicating with caregivers and loved ones. In later stages, the individual may not be able to speak coherently and may become unresponsive to most (or any) stimuli. Caregivers can follow these steps to ensure that the person in a later stage of dementia still receives a high quality of care.

Checklist: Tips for the caregiver when the individual enters the later stages of dementia

- [ ] Ensure that the individual has a living space that is familiar and safe. Make the space as cheery as possible. For example, a suncatcher in a window can not only help brighten the living space, but it can give you clues as to the individual's level of responsiveness to external stimuli.

- [ ] It is very likely that when the individual enters the later stages of dementia you will need to take the individual's car keys away—if you have not already done that. Although it can be painful to do this because of the taking away of one of the last vestiges of the individual's freedom this represents, the individual's safety needs to come first.

- [ ] Monitor the individual's total physical and emotional health and ensure that appropriate medical intervention is provided if and when necessary. Ensure that other conditions are treated so dementia does not exacerbate them. You can schedule visits with relatives and friends as well as meal services and other support services through Caring Bridge.

- [ ] Beyond medical interventions, ensure that the individual's daily comfort is being provided for as much as possible. Ensure that the individual is kept clean with proper maintenance of hygiene. Ensure that bedsheets and clothing are changed regularly.

- [ ] It might be helpful to make a list of your loved one's habits and schedule as well as things that calm or distress your loved one so that others can do the things that are most beneficial for your loved one and avoid what has proven not to be helpful.

- [ ] Emphasize your loved one's individuality to all non-primary caregivers.

- [ ] Acknowledge that all the individual's behaviors are meaningful and represent an impulse to communicate. This is true even of acting out, which often is a sign of pain or distress and a clue that you should attempt to find out what's wrong. When the individual attempts to speak or otherwise be understood, provide a response, even if it's just a steady gaze and smile while holding the individual's hand.

☐ Keep yourself mentally and physically healthy so that you can provide high-quality, emotionally competent care. Particularly in the later stages, your wellness is closely linked with the wellness of your loved one.

In addition to adult caregivers, young people may interact with the individual with dementia. Children and teenagers may not understand the emotional needs of the individual with dementia. They may emphasize their own feelings about the diagnosis. Young children might express fear that they will get dementia or that they may have caused it. Teens might become resentful if they have to assume extra responsibility or may experience embarrassment. College-age young people might be hesitant to be away from home or feel the need to stay away.

Checklist: Considerations to help children adjust

☐ Discuss the disease with children openly, especially when they ask about the individual's condition. Providing context can be essential to helping them understand the changes the individual is going through.

☐ Discover the child's emotional needs and find ways to support them as they come to terms with the condition. Meeting with a therapist can be a helpful step in addressing a child's emotional health.

☐ If you are close to a particular child or your situation might directly affect them, discuss the situation with school officials and classroom teachers.

☐ Educate children about dementia and the changes that it is creating in their family.

☐ Lighten the mood with humor. The situation is distressing, but with humor you can help reduce the burden of coping.

It's easy, in the process of caregiving, for caregivers to overlook their own needs. The following section examines what caregivers need to do themselves to avoid burnout and other health problems that can develop from the burden of caregiving.

Emotional Considerations for the Caregiver

Caregivers for individuals with dementia are doubly vulnerable to deep and confusing emotions: they have to come to terms with a loved one's diagnosis while providing draining and stressful day-to-day care over the course of the illness. As a caregiver, you are susceptible to a wide range of stress-related issues, particularly as the disease enters the moderate to severe stages and the demands on you increase in number and intensity. As a first step, you should learn as much as possible about the condition. By recognizing which elements of the disease can be changed, caregivers can set their expectations appropriately to accept what they cannot change. You should also identify sources of help, such as local services, adult care, and respite services, to know where to turn when you can't give any more.

Watching my father decline left me in a state of depression that was paralyzing at times. I tried talking to people about it, but they just didn't seem to understand, and I personally found support groups to be more depressing. Once dad was in a nursing home, the two things I did to help were to cut back on the number of times I saw dad per week and to start writing short stories. The writing gave me a creative outlet that was cheaper than therapy. What works for you may be different, but try to find an activity that gives you an emotional outlet that doesn't force you to dwell on the sadness.

All Caregivers

All caregivers need to find ways to cope with their emotions, maintain a positive attitude, and reduce their stress and anxiety. Above all, they must ensure that in giving care they also care for themselves. You can't help others if you burn yourself out by refusing to recognize and properly deal with your own physical and emotional stressors.

Managing Emotions

The constant strain of caregiving can have a broad range of negative effects on your physical and mental health as well as the well-being of your loved one and your family. One thing that helped me (Laura) was taking a break and not seeing my dad for a couple of weeks when he was in the nursing home. I only did this two to three times a year, but it helped tremendously. Getting some distance helped me regain some perspective. If you are caregiving full time, ask friends or hire home health care to come in so you can take a break. Another thing that helped was planning something I would enjoy every week so I had something to look forward to. Do what works for you to keep yourself going. The following checklist examines many of these negative effects and useful strategies for mitigating them.

Checklist: How to manage negative effects of caregiving

Denial:

- [ ] Denial is understandable at first in processing the news that a loved one has been diagnosed with dementia. However, acknowledge that although some fear about the future is inevitable, it is not in your loved one's best interest to deny that the diagnosis is real or that the symptoms are serious.

- [ ] To get past your emotional impulse to deny the reality of your loved one's illness, think of what a rational response to the situation would be. Objectively, without your own emotions as a factor and focusing as much as possible on facts, what is your loved one's situation? What does your loved one need most from you?

- [ ] Realize that inaction rooted in denial is a kind of action. The loved one who has been diagnosed with dementia will be in even deeper denial than you. By helping them work through their emotions, you can work on your own.

- [ ] Similarly, helping family members in denial understand that it is in everyone's best interest to fully acknowledge the significance of the disease can help you do so yourself.

Frustration and Guilt:

☐ Feelings of frustration and guilt are inevitable. You will not be able to do all that you want to do, and as the pressures of the disease mount and your loved one's condition deteriorates, your frustration is likely to be unmanageable sometimes. That is likely to make you feel guilty. This is normal. Don't beat yourself up.

☐ Remember that you have limited control over the situation and should not feel guilty when you reach the end of your ability to help your loved one. No one expects you to be a professionally trained caregiver, and there will come a time when your loved one's needs are greater than your skills. Have a plan in place for what to do when this happens.

☐ Seek out help when you feel overwhelmed by your lack of ability to help your loved one and when you feel that your control over your own emotions about the situation is slipping.

☐ Caregiving is hard, and you will often hate it. It can seem to have no end and no reward. It can be boring or mind numbing. When you feel guilty about these natural feelings, remind yourself that caregiving does have a purpose, even if it is difficult to see. Your loved one depends on everything you do, and it matters.

☐ You should never feel guilty about enjoying time to yourself or with family and friends, pursuing your own interests, and generally living your own life. You need to do what you can for your loved one, but you need to have a life too to maintain your own emotional health.

Anger and Resentment:

☐ Your daily life will be significantly affected by the duties of caregiving. This can cause resentment and even anger to build, and at time these feelings can seem uncontrollable. To handle anger and resentment, first recognize that you are feeling them. Be honest with yourself, but also recognize that feelings such as these are natural.

☐ Count to ten. It's very simple, but when you feel the anger and resentment building, you first need to refuse to be a channel for it. Take a step back from what you're feeling when you think you might be losing control. Not being a channel for these feelings includes not participating in activities that enable you to wallow in the anger and resentment. This may seem like venting, but it can actually fuel these feelings. You do need to talk to others about how you are feeling, but always to acknowledge it and then look for ways past it.

☐ What causes or worsens the anger and resentment? If you recognize tasks or situations that can cause your anger and resentment to flare up, you can be prepared for it.

☐ Observe how you act when you give in to the anger and resentment. What do these emotions cause you to do? How do you release that emotion on the person with dementia and on others? Find a different way to express those feelings that has positive results, such as going for a run, playing a sport, writing in a journal, or something else that allows you to channel that negative energy into something positive.

☐ Form the habit of looking at every difficult situation from another person's standpoint: the person with dementia, others providing care, other loved ones. What do they feel? What do they need? Because it can be easy to lose these thoughts when you are in the grip of emotions such as anger and resentment, practice this mindfulness as a matter of routine as a way of starving those negative emotions of the fuel they need to exist.

☐ It can seem impossible to do this at this time, but practice feeling grateful. List and remember all that you have to feel grateful for. Keep a gratitude journal. Practicing gratitude is like practicing empathy: Make it a part of your routine.

Always remember the abundant blessings in your life because these can lift you up when you need it the most.

Depression:

☐ Depression can take many forms, but in all cases it is a destructive mood disorder that significantly interferes with your ability to be satisfied with your life. Depression often affects basic needs, such as sleep or hunger, but it doesn't

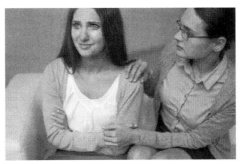
Credit: Pressmaster

always affect them the same way for every individual. Consider seeking treatment for depression if you experience these symptoms a significant amount of the time:

- Loss of interest in or inability to derive pleasure from activities that normally would give you pleasure

- An inability to sleep or sleeping too much

- A loss of appetite and desire to eat or eating too much

- Abnormally slowed thinking and responses or agitation and restlessness

- Frequent outbursts, anger, and frustration, even if the current situation shouldn't provoke such responses

- Loss of concentration and focus and feelings of tiredness and helplessness

- Thoughts of death and suicide

- Physical problems with no apparent cause

☐ Because the effects of depression can mimic those of other conditions, it can be difficult to know sometimes that depression is the reason you are experiencing these problems.

Generally, though, if you have a persistent downturn in mood that seriously conflicts with your ability to function in a normal way, and especially if this persistent mood causes you to contemplate suicide, seek medical help.

☐ Your doctor can rule out depression as a cause for your symptoms if they have another cause. If you are depressed, your doctor can refer you to an appropriate mental health specialist or provide you with medication as necessary.

☐ Try to keep in contact with friends and family, take breaks, exercise, and eat a balanced diet. Depression tends to interfere with all of these activities, so it can be difficult to manage if you are severely depressed, but try.

☐ Medications, if appropriate for your needs, can lift your mood, though they may not take full effect for six to eight weeks.

☐ Counseling with a mental health specialist, such as a psychiatrist, clinical psychologist, social worker, or licensed mental health counselor, can be very effective in treating depression.

☐ Developing individual coping skills is a necessary part of managing depression as well. Learning relaxation and stress relief methods as well as expressive strategies such as journaling can help you manage your mood.

☐ Avoid drug and alcohol use, which can exacerbate the problems of mood disorders.

☐ Remember that depression isn't typically something you can simply snap out of. It's a persistent medical condition that typically requires professional intervention to treat. Don't try to go it alone.

Anxiety:

☐ Anxiety disorder is not worrying sometimes about problems. It is intense and excessive worry that persists even in everyday situations that should not provoke such an emotional reaction. Anxiety disorder interferes with a person's ability to function on a daily basis. Symptoms of anxiety disorder include:

- A sense of impending danger or doom

- A feeling of tension, nervousness, or restlessness

- Increased heart rate and rapid breathing with sweating and trembling

- Persistent fixation on the feeling of worry

- Trouble sleeping and a feeling of fatigue or weakness

- Gastrointestinal problems

- Avoidance of known triggers for anxiety

☐ A persistent sense of worry may be related to identifiable and ongoing stressors, such as money worries, difficulty finding work, etc. If this is the case, then addressing the stressor should address the worry; for example, getting help from family members in paying your bills while you provide care should help relieve financial stress. However, if you can't identify a specific stressor that causes your anxiety or you address all known stressors and your anxiety persists, then you likely have an anxiety disorder.

☐ Visit your doctor right away if you believe you have an anxiety disorder. Your physician will be able to prescribe medication, as appropriate, or refer you to a mental health professional.

☐ Try to stay active and focused on identifiable problems. Caregiving actually can help with that by giving you something to focus on that requires specific interventions.

☐ When you become overwhelmed by the responsibilities of caregiving and are experiencing strong anxiety, use relaxation techniques, such as focused deep breathing or guided imagery, to provide short-term relief. See the checklist on relaxation methods later in this book for some examples of what you can do.

- Avoid drug and alcohol use, which can exacerbate the problems of mood disorders.

Exhaustion and Discouragement:

- Spend time with friends and family to ensure that you still have a regular source of social interaction. Even if you are completely exhausted after caregiving, ensure that you still share experiences with others to reduce the chronic strain of caregiving.

- Reach out to caregiving organizations for education and support, look for resources in your community, investigate commercial elder care businesses such as respite care centers, and take time for yourself.

- When you reach the limits of your physical and mental ability to cope, make an effort to take pressure off yourself.

- Ask family members to help with elements of care, such as grocery shopping, doing laundry, cleaning, or even just spending time with the individual with dementia.

- Hire outside help, if feasible, to provide in-home care or adult daycare.

- Take breaks periodically to ensure that you are not working yourself to exhaustion.

- When the person with dementia doesn't cooperate or the caregiver comes to realize that there is yet another thing the individual can no longer do on their own, the weight on the caregiver just gets heavier and heavier, which can be enormously discouraging. When you begin to feel this, and whenever you become exhausted to the point that you feel you can't go on, accept help, and

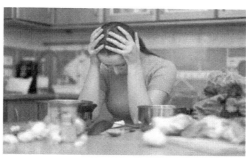
Credit: Iakov Filimonov

22

don't be afraid to ask for assistance. You'll feel better supported, and your relationships with your family and friends will grow stronger in the process. Don't just keep going it alone! Always reach out, for your well-being and the individual's.

Sleep Problems:

- ☐ If you are sleeping poorly or too much, make solving your chronic tiredness a priority. Quality sleep is essential to mental and physical wellness.

- ☐ If you consume caffeine or alcohol close to bedtime and commonly experience sleep disturbances, consider cutting down on your consumption of these substances, especially in the evening, to regulate your sleeping patterns.

- ☐ Stress and anxiety are contributing factors to sleep disturbances. Take the steps outlined in this book to reduce the effects of stress and anxiety on your life.

- ☐ If your sleep problems persist, see a doctor. Your physician will be able to help you keep track of your sleep disturbances and work with you to change problematic behaviors.

Illness:

- ☐ The constant stress of being a caregiver can contribute significantly to your risk of developing a short-term or chronic health condition.

- ☐ Watch your diet and ensure that you are eating a healthy balance of foods.

- ☐ Take time to exercise regularly. A caregiver's time is in short supply, but you don't need to buy a gym membership and talk to a personal trainer. Try to spend 20 or 30 minutes every day walking or doing yoga to start.

- ☐ If you smoke, stop. Smoking increases your susceptibility to illnesses of all kinds.

- ☐ Take steps to get a good night's sleep.

☐ Take the steps listed in this section to reduce stress, anxiety, and depression.

Grief

Everyone is familiar with the idea of grief following the death of a loved one or a loved one being diagnosed with a terminal illness. But people also can experience grief if they have an illness for which there is no cure, although it is not life threatening, or a chronic condition that affects their quality of life. Grief concerns loss, and not necessarily loss of life; it could be loss of independence, loss of physical or cognitive function, or anything else the grieving person values that is diminishing or gone. Grief that occurs before a significant loss is called anticipatory grief.

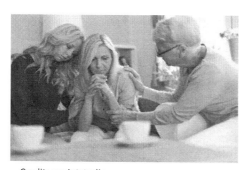
Credit: gpointstudio

Everyone feels grief in their own way. There are, however, common stages in the process of mourning. People's responses to grief from the death of a loved one will be different, depending on the circumstances of the death. In the case of grieving for someone with dementia, family and friends of the person with the disease may experience different stages of grief before and after the person passes away, depending on their personality and relationship with the person with the condition. The pain of anticipatory grief is often compounded not only by the responsibilities of caregiving and the exhaustion of managing the symptoms of dementia but also by the way that the progression of the disease takes away more and more of the person the loved one once was with the passage of time.

Grief is frequently described in five stages. These reactions might not occur in a specific order, and they can occur together. Not everyone experiences all of these emotions.

Checklist: The stages of grief

- ☐ Denial, disbelief, numbness

- ☐ Anger, blaming others

- ☐ Bargaining

- ☐ Depressed mood, sadness, and crying

- ☐ Acceptance, coming to terms

Grief is a healthy response to loss and should not be stifled, but the sadness and anger associated with this feeling can become overwhelming. People who are grieving may have crying spells, trouble sleeping, and lack of productivity at work. There is no "correct" way to respond to loss, no normal timetable for grieving, and no easily defined grieving process.

Checklist: Managing grief

- ☐ To begin managing grief, talk to family and friends. They can offer emotional support during the grieving process. Express your feelings as a way of exploring them in a way that you find productive.

- ☐ See a health care provider or grief counselor. These professionals can help place your loss in context and provide you with strategies you can use to manage your feelings.

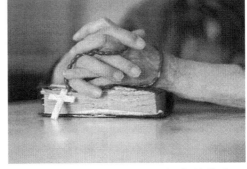

- ☐ Join a support group in which members share common experiences and problems to help relieve the stress from grieving.

Credit: Halfpoint

- ☐ If you take part in a religious or spiritual tradition, participate in religious rituals to gain comfort and confidence in something outside yourself. Talking with clergy about your loss can be a source of comfort.

- Write in a journal about your feelings, make a scrapbook, or get involved in an activity that is or was important to the person you are grieving.

- Stay physically healthy to lift your mood. Eat well, exercise regularly, and don't use drugs and alcohol excessively.

- Connect with loved ones, but if people judge the way that you are grieving, don't feel shame or embarrassment about what is natural for you. It can be hard to take when people tell you to "get over it" when you know you are not at a point that you can let your grief go. Just remember that there is no set timetable for emotions such as grief. You need to process your feelings in your own way and your own time.

- However, distinct from normal grieving, which leads to eventual acceptance, complicated grief, which impedes healing, can be a problem. Complicated grief is marked by a prolonged intensity of sorrow over and fixation on the loss in a way that produces much the same effect as severe depression. In complicated grief, the person is inconsolable and clings to the loss, which becomes all that matters to the person. You need to work through your grief in your own time, but if after months you are not moving toward healing, consider that you may have complicated grief and seek professional help to work through your feelings.

- Be aware of grief "triggers," such as holidays, birthdays, and family milestones, as these events may produce unusually strong grief reactions.

The long-term strain of being an dementia caregiver can lead to a feeling of being trapped in a hopeless situation with no way out. Because people with dementia progressively decline in mental and physical function, caregiving can become harder with time, not easier. The task of caregiving can stretch on for years. This can come to seem intolerable. For some caregivers, suicide may seem like a way out. The problems that commonly accompany caregiving for a person with a terminal illness, such as depression, anxiety, and prolonged stress, are also some of the risk factors for suicide. Be aware of these risks and how to prevent them. (For a more detailed discussion of suicide risks and prevention in the context of dementia, see the section on suicide in *Home Safety Checklist Guide and Caregiver Resources for Medication Safety, Driving, and Wandering.*)

Checklist: Suicide risk and prevention

- ☐ Risk factors for suicide include:

    - Depression

    - Mood and personality disorders

    - Substance abuse

    - Impulsiveness

    - An inability to solve problems

    - Hopelessness

    - Social isolation

    - Thinking about suicide as a way out

    - A family history of suicide or a personal history of previous suicide attempts

- ☐ Prevention of suicide involves treating the underlying problems that can lead to suicide risk. Identify your specific suicide risk factors—depression, anxiety, stress, and so on— and seek treatment for those problems. Many of the resources in this book can help get you started on coping with some of the problems that can pose a risk for suicide.

- ☐ A risk factor for suicide is simply access to the means to do it. Assess your environment for potential means for suicide and then try as much as possible to remove those means if you think you are at risk.

- ☐ Talk to others about your feelings. Don't stay isolated and alone. Reach out to others for support. Talk to professionals.

- ☐ A mental health provider can provide you with specific treatment options tailored to your particular needs, including medication and counseling.

- ☐ If you are prone to substance abuse, remember that substance abuse is a risk factor for suicide, not a way out. If you need treatment for substance abuse, be honest with yourself about that need and seek help. You can't care for others if you don't provide yourself with the care you need first.

- ☐ If you are having suicidal intentions or thoughts, get in touch with a medical professional or suicide hotline as quickly as possible. Call 800-SUICIDE (800-784-2433) or 800-273-TALK (800-273-8255) or the deaf hotline at 800-799-4889.

Reducing Stress

Caregivers are tasked with a lot of responsibilities: overseeing medical services, transportation, and household responsibilities, all while dealing with the emotional aspects of the prolonged loss of a loved one. The pressure can be overwhelming, but caregivers can make their task easier, which can contribute to lower stress and healthier outcomes.

Checklist: Basics about managing your role as a caregiver

- ☐ Research dementia to know what to expect over the course of the disease. Read as much as possible and talk with other caregivers to discover research related to prevention and treatment options.

- ☐ Let go of unrealistic expectations surrounding dementia. The condition is terminal, and the reality is that the loved one's gradual memory loss and need for more intensive care are inevitable. You can help improve your loved one's quality of life, but their illness is ultimately out of your hands.

- ☐ Locate resources that can help you. Seek out government and community services such as adult day care and respite services, and contact them as needed to reduce the stress of supporting someone with dementia.

- ☐ When your loved one becomes confused, reassure them rather than employing confrontation. When your loved one suffers delusions and acts strangely, gently redirect them toward a more realistic line of thought or productive task rather than chastising them. If necessary, set the task aside for later, and you might need to reassess whether your loved one can perform the task in question at all. Be realistic for your loved one's sake and for your own.

☐ Construct a predictable and reassuring environment for yourself and the person with dementia by establishing a simple daily routine. Look into resources on home safety for people with dementia.

☐ Plan for legal and financial issues as soon as possible. Gather necessary legal and financial documents so that your loved one can make as many decisions as possible, or at least so that legal and financial decisions do not add stress to the caregiving process later.

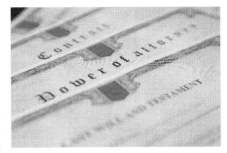
Credit: NotarYES

☐ Keep in mind that your relationship with your loved one will evolve over time. Family roles will change, and you might be placed in charge of activities that you may not feel entirely capable of handling. Your loved one will slowly lose the ability to perform their old roles within the family.

☐ You ultimately only have control over your own responses and attitudes. You can't control what happens, only how you react to it. Practice positive self-talk to cultivate a positive attitude.

☐ Trust in your ability as a caregiver. Many times, your instincts can lead you in the right direction.

You will most effectively reduce stress if you simultaneously lessen the impact of stressors in your life and increase your ability to cope with them. Lessening the impact of stressors can be accomplished by understanding your role as a caregiver and attempting to manage it. Coping with stress can be accomplished through the following steps for emotional management. One major thing to keep in mind is that you will have setbacks. Don't beat yourself up when that happens. This is a process. Take joy in the progress you make, but if there's a slip in that progress and you let the stress get to you, that's okay. Just keep doing what you can to minimize the number and impact of stressors in your life while maximizing your ability to cope with them.

Checklist: Basics about reducing stress

☐ Take a break from your responsibilities for ten to twenty minutes a day and spend time in meditation or reflection. The form of your meditation can be aligned with a spiritual tradition, but it doesn't have to be. It can be as simple as taking a few moments to slow down your thoughts.

☐ Exercise to pour your energy into something other than your problems as well as benefit your mind and body. Aerobic exercise involves the heart, lungs, and blood flow. Repeatedly moving large muscles increases the rapidity and depth of your breathing, increasing the amount of oxygen in your blood. Additionally, your heart beats faster, which increases blood flow. Some examples of aerobic exercise:

- Walking

- Running or jogging

- Bicycling

- Swimming

- Dancing

- Jumping rope

☐ Some benefits of aerobic exercise in addition to elevating your mood:

- Lose weight.

- Increase endurance and strength.

- Strengthen your heart and keep your arteries clear.

- Extend your independence as you age and lengthen your life expectancy.

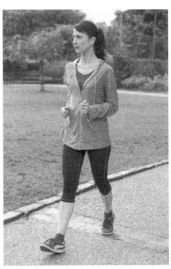
Credit: Image Point Fr

□ See your doctor regularly and maintain your physical health. Physical well-being is closely tied to emotional health.

□ Keep active with hobbies that involve your mind and/or body, such as gardening, playing or listening to music, knitting, cooking, or reading. Having hobbies outside your role as a caregiver ensures that you still have an independent life and sense of self-worth.

□ Make to-do lists to keep track of your upcoming responsibilities. Calendars and planners can help you survey your priorities at a glance.

□ Avoid stressful multitasking and try to streamline your caregiving tasks. Trying to do too much at once just adds to your stress level.

□ Understand the limits of your role as caregiver, and don't be afraid to say "no." If you are emotionally spent, you will not be able to provide high-quality care.

□ Talk to friends and family regularly to have partners in coping. No one is emotionally capable of being a caregiver alone. Talk about your problems as a way of sorting them out.

□ Write your thoughts out in a journal to gain a nuanced understanding of your emotions. Writing feelings down can provide clarity in confusing situations.

□ Use humor to lighten the situations you find yourself in as a caregiver. Seek out funny books and movies as a way of lifting your mood.

☐ When good things happen, appreciate them. Be open to moments of pleasure, such as small moments with your loved one, visits with family members, and simple activities like a walk in springtime.

☐ Appreciate that you are doing a very hard job. Caring for someone with dementia is often a thankless task, but you should allow yourself to feel a sense of accomplishment.

☐ Pay attention to what you are learning from the process of caregiving. Appreciate your growing wisdom and what you have accomplished that you would not have thought possible.

Taking care of yourself is one of your most important responsibilities as a caregiver. This could mean asking family members or friends to help out, engaging in activities you enjoy, using adult day care services, or getting help from a local home health care agency. Taking these actions can bring you some relief. It also may help keep you from getting ill or depressed.

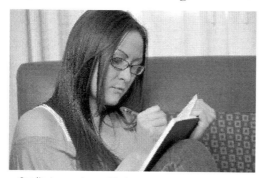
Credit: Image Aspen Photo

Checklist: Basics about maintaining a positive attitude

☐ Ask for help when you need it.

☐ Join a caregivers' support group.

☐ Take breaks each day.

☐ Spend time with friends.

☐ Keep up with your hobbies and interests.

☐ Eat healthy foods.

☐ Get exercise as often as you can.

☐ See your doctor on a regular basis.

☐ Keep your health, legal, and financial information up to date.

An important component of maintaining a positive attitude is engaging in positive self-talk. Consistently framing events and thoughts in positive terms can reshape your thought processes so that you tend to naturally think in a positive frame of mind.

Checklist: Basics about practicing positive self-talk

☐ Identify negative thoughts that arise in relation to your caregiving responsibilities. For example, "No one ever thanks me for my work" is a negative thought that can lead to negative emotions.

☐ Is there a rational basis for the negative thought? If so, is there something you can change? For example, if the thought is "No one ever thanks me for my work," and you really can't think of examples where anyone has thanked you for the things you do, then think about whether that is something you can address with the people who are in your primary emotional support group.

☐ If you don't see an easy solution for the negative thought, and especially if there isn't really a rational basis for the thought, actively replace the negative thought with a positive version. For example, "No one ever thanks me for my work" could become "I am the best person for this job."

☐ Replacing the negative thought with a positive version should be easiest when a little reflection reveals that the negative thought isn't entirely rational. For example, if you reflect on the thought "No one ever thanks me for my work" and realize that in fact people do thank you, that you're just having a bad day, the positive thought is easy: "People recognize and are grateful for the work that I do."

☐ These modified thoughts displace the steady stream of negativity, in the process replacing emotions such as anger, frustration, and guilt with hope, empowerment, and humor.

- Positive self-talk should not be a way of glossing over real problems. If a negative thought involves something that requires real attention, then positive self-talk should not take the place of actively addressing that problem. But positive self-talk can help you keep your spirits up and not take things so hard when you're having a bad day and feeling overwhelmed.

Another way to promote a positive attitude is to practice relaxation techniques. Relaxation techniques include practices such as progressive relaxation, guided imagery, biofeedback, self-hypnosis, and deep breathing exercises. The goal is similar in all: to produce the body's natural relaxation response, characterized by slower breathing, lower blood pressure, and a feeling of increased well-being. Meditation and practices that combine meditation with movement, such as yoga and tai chi, can also promote relaxation. Stress management programs commonly include relaxation techniques. Relaxation techniques have also been studied to see whether they might be of value in managing various health problems. Different techniques work for different people. If one technique doesn't click with you, try another until you find something that really does help you relax.

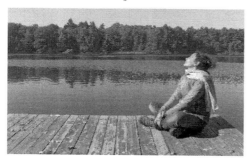

Credit: Image ArTono

Checklist: Basics about relaxation techniques

- Autogenic training was invented by a psychiatrist, Johannes Heinrich Schultz, in 1932. It consists of progressive relaxation of the extremities, stabilization of the heartbeat, and maintenance of slow, deep breathing.

  - In autogenic relaxation, you first find a comfortable position.

  - A therapist instructs you to focus on different parts of your body and relax your breathing.

- Sessions involve promoting awareness of specific parts of your body and concentrating in various ways: inducing heaviness and feelings of warmth, focusing on the heartbeat and abdominal sensations, regulating breathing, feeling coolness on the forehead.

- The therapist uses verbal cues, such as "My left leg is heavy" or "My heartbeat is calm and steady," to promote this concentration on specific aspects of specific areas.

- You must commit to performing autogenic exercises at least once daily. This type of training requires sustained commitment to work.

- Benefits of autogenic training include reduced stress and anxiety.

- Deep breathing exercises involves taking slow, deep, even breaths, which sends a message to your brain to relax.

  - A basic type of deep breathing exercise is called belly breathing. To begin belly breathing, first find a comfortable position to sit or lie flat.

  - Place one hand on your belly just below your ribs. Place the other hand on your chest.

  - Breathe in deeply through your nose and let your belly push your hand out without moving your chest.

  - Breathe out through pursed lips while using your belly hand to push all the air out.

  - Do this three to ten times. Take your time.

  - 4-7-8 breathing is a type of belly breathing in which you draw in your breath for 4 seconds, hold it for 7 seconds, and then release it for 8 seconds.

  - Other types of deep breathing are roll breathing and morning breathing.

- Doing these exercises helps you relax, relieves stress, and reduces tension.

☐ The guided imagery technique involves focusing on pleasant images to replace negative or stressful feelings.

- Guided imagery may be self-directed or led by a practitioner or a recording.

- Guided imagery takes many forms, but it fundamentally involves using the imagination to actively visualize calming, peaceful images. Instead of going somewhere peaceful, your imagination creates that place within you.

- Scripts can guide this technique, and aids such as soothing music can be helpful.

- Guided imagery can decrease depression, stress, and anxiety while increasing sleep and relaxation and enhancing quality of life.

☐ Investigate the progressive relaxation technique, also called Jacobson relaxation or progressive muscle relaxation, which involves tightening and relaxing various muscle groups.

- Progressive relaxation is often combined with guided imagery and breathing exercises.

- One method involves beginning with tensing and relaxing your toe muscles and then working your way up to your neck and head. You can also reverse this process by beginning with your head and neck and then working your way down to your toes.

- Tension of the muscles should be about 5 seconds followed by relaxation for about 30 seconds, then repeat.

- Progressive relaxation has many benefits, including improved concentration and mood, decreased fatigue and stress, and improved sleep quality and digestion.

☐ Other techniques for relaxation include massage, meditation, Tai chi, yoga, biofeedback, music and art therapy, aromatherapy, and hydrotherapy. This list has described some of the more common methods for relaxation, but with so many options to explore, don't give up until you find a technique that works best for you.

Maintaining Communication

Frequent communication with others who are involved in caregiving along with you is fundamental to maintaining emotional health and a sense of perspective while providing care to an individual with dementia. One of the best ways to educate yourself about dementia while relieving the stress of caregiving is to communicate with your support network and other caregivers. Keeping in touch with a strong support network can keep you sane by allowing you to express your feelings and hear others' points of view, receive empathy from others who are going or have gone through the same thing, educate you by exposing you to new points of view, and provide you with a community of people who can provide help in times of need.

Checklist: Basics about communicating with your support network and other caregivers

☐ Communicate regularly with your family and friends about your role as a caregiver. Communicating with your relatives is particularly important: They also have a stake in your loved one's health, even if they are not the primary caregivers.

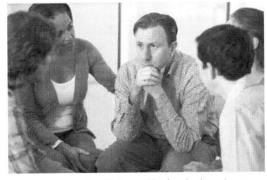

☐ Accept help when family and friends offer it. Bringing your loved ones into the caregiving process can help them understand

Credit: Image Monkey Business Images

your responsibilities and point of view.

- Don't be afraid to talk to friends and loved ones about the serious aspects of caregiving, including your fears and the parts of the caregiving process that intimidate you.

- Join a formal support group, such as one offered by a church or an organization such as the Alzheimer's Association. These organizations can enable you to bond with caregivers in positions similar to yours. Every group has a different dynamic, some you will respond to and others you won't. I (Laura) never found a group I connected with, but I have friends who found them invaluable.

- Join an online support group, such as ElderCare Online's Caregiver Support Network or the Alzheimer's Association's AlzConnected. These services offer online discussion groups, forums, social groups, and resource lists that can help you feel connected in your caregiving.

The time pressures and emotional strain of providing full-time care can be overwhelming. Maintaining your friendships and other relationships throughout the disease process is essential to doing the best you can during the difficult times. Ensure that you continue to put energy toward the other people in your life.

Checklist: How to maintain friendships and other relationships

- As a caregiver, much of your attention is lavished on one person, and it's easy to let that narrow focus become your entire world. Remember to take a step back from your caregiver role to connect with the other people in your life.

- To ensure that you can stay close with other friends and family throughout the caregiving process, review the relationships that are important to you and remember to pay particularly close attention to maintaining those.

- Consistently communicate and establish rituals with loved ones. Designate particular times to perform different activities with loved ones.

- Ensure that you continue listening to friends' problems, no matter how seemingly trivial. Your life as a caregiver is doubtless full of strong emotions and dramatic moments, and you will want to share those with your loved ones, but your relationships cannot thrive over the long run if they are one sided. You may find it to be a refreshing change of pace if other people talk to you about the small stuff. Maybe you should too.

☐ Be careful to share appropriate amounts of information about your work as a caregiver. Your friends and family should be willing to hear your concerns, but all relationships need give and take if everyone is to feel good about them.

☐ Realize that others will have a hard time relating to your issue. The work of a caregiver is difficult for a non-caregiver to understand, particularly if they have a different relationship with your loved one with dementia.

☐ Accept disagreements and resolve them the best you can. Your family and friends will sometimes disagree with caregiving decisions or even be in denial about certain aspects of your loved one's diagnosis. Compromise when possible, and consider using a family mediator when disagreements become heated.

☐ Some relationships might fall by the wayside. For example, tangential friends or relatives who are not close to you or the individual with dementia might argue with decisions made in the best interest of that person. In such cases, it may be best to put these relationships on the back burner or cut them off entirely if they become a stressor or get in the way of more meaningful relationships.

Maintaining Health

Caregiving can take an overwhelming amount of time, and frequently one of the first necessities to be neglected is physical health. Emotional health and physical health are closely tied, so be sure to support your ability to cope by keeping yourself fit.

☐ Try to plan at least one activity a week that you can look forward to. It might be something as simple as going to lunch with a friend or watching a movie, but it will give you something positive to focus on.

☐ Visit the doctor regularly (at least once a year) to ensure that you're in good health. Pay close attention to any physical symptoms; ignoring your body's messages can cause your health to decline.

☐ Exercise regularly to relieve stress, prevent illness, and improve your mood. To find time to exercise, take advantage of moments when others take over caregiving responsibilities to work out at home and perform an exercise activity that you enjoy doing.

☐ To benefit both you and your loved one with dementia, take part in physical exercise together. Walk together outside, exercise at home, or dance together. These kinds of exercise also serve as a way of keeping close with your loved one.

☐ Eat a balanced diet rich in a wide variety of nutrients, but don't eat to excess. A Mediterranean diet, an eating pattern that emphasizes healthy fats, fruits, vegetables, nuts, fish, and grains, is currently recommended by doctors.

Ensuring Proper Care in a Facility

Emotional considerations for the caregiver may extend beyond the stage of direct caregiving. If your loved one is in a long-term care facility and you do not directly provide day-to-day care, you might be anxious about the quality of care they are receiving, especially because you are no longer the person giving it. Letting this responsibility go to others can be difficult, but you still have a job to do, and it is still to ensure your loved one is receiving proper and necessary care.

Years ago, before my father was sick, I (Laura) volunteered in nursing homes and would visit people who did not have any family or friends. I often learned that the patients did have family or friends—or at least, they did when they were healthy—but that those people had abandoned them. Every week, I would get very angry about this. When my dad got sick, I had a close friend tell me not to visit him because life is for the living and dad was essentially dead. I largely ignored this advice, but I learned two things from it. The first one was that it is different watching your own loved ones decline and visiting them than it is strangers. It is much harder to visit a loved one than it is to be a volunteer and visit strangers. You have memories and expectations with your loved one. You expect your father to know his name or understand what a mirror is. You do not have the same expectations with strangers. The second, and more important, lesson I learned is that I didn't have to visit every day. I felt like being a good daughter was visiting every day, but it became too depressing. I had two young children, and being sandwiched between their needs and what I perceived to be dad's needs to be was difficult. Once I allowed myself not to visit every single day, I was able to be a better mother to my children, and I cherished the time with my father more. It also helped that by this time, dad had no awareness of whether I was there or not, so I knew that my visits did not affect his mental state. What my visits did do, however, was make sure that staff were keeping an eye on him and being responsive. They often were not responsive. I think this is true in every nursing home, and it's a crisis in this country. Nursing homes are in the business to make a profit, and they will hire the fewest number of people they can for the least amount of pay that they can. Nurses and nursing assistants are given an overwhelming workload, while the patients are paying thousands of dollars a month for substandard care. So even while your loved one may not know whether you visit or not, it's still good to visit unannounced, outside a normal schedule, so you can be a healthcare advocate.

Checklist: How to ensure proper care is being given in a facility

☐ Tour assisted living or long-term care facilities before there is any immediate pressure to move so that you make a good decision when the time comes. (For more information on living arrangements, see *Home Care, Long-term Care, Memory Care Units, and Other Living Arrangements*).

☐ Check for signs of physical abuse, such as unexplained injuries, apparent failure to take medication regularly, signs of being restrained, or the caregiver's refusal to allow you to see your loved one alone.

☐ Check for signs of emotional abuse, such as threatening or controlling caregiver behavior or emotional distress on your loved one's part.

☐ Check for signs of sexual abuse, including bruises or bleeding around genitals, unexplained STDs, or torn or stained underclothing.

☐ Check for signs of neglect, including unexplained weight loss, untreated physical problems, unsanitary conditions, and abandonment of your loved one in public.

☐ Check for signs of financial exploitation, including duplicate billings, overmedication, inadequate care, and issues with the care facility.

☐ Listen to your loved one if they mention any potentially abusive behaviors and then follow up to investigate these claims.

☐ Regularly visit the long-term care facility and personally check that conditions are adequate.

☐ If you think that your loved one is suffering from inadequate conditions or elder abuse in a full-time care facility, file a complaint with your state health agency. The state will contact you within a few days and send an agent for a surprise visit to the care facility. See the Resources at the end of this chapter for more information on reporting nursing home abuse.

☐ Also send a copy of your complaint to your state's Association for the Protection of the Elderly (APE). These organizations ensure that the state adequately investigates your complaint.

☐ For faster and more direct action, contact a lawyer to file legal action directly against the care facility that is committing elder abuse.

Spouses

If your spouse has dementia, the marital roles in your relationship will change as the disease progresses. Ask for help as you take on new responsibilities, such as paying bills, that you may not have had to handle before. You will experience changes in emotional and sexual intimacy as well as having to cope with grief as the disease progresses. Try whenever possible to spend time together with your spouse in ways that you both find fulfilling and that bring you closer together. Reach out to others for emotional support whenever you need it.

Checklist: Basics about changing marital roles

- ☐ You may have to take on tasks that are unfamiliar to you, such as cooking, doing chores, and handling financial and legal matters.

- ☐ As you learn new skills, be sure to ask for help when you need it. Family members and friends may be able to help you cope with your new role and even take on some responsibility.

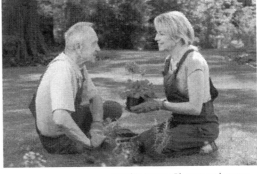
Credit: Image Photographee.eu

- ☐ If you are taking on financial and legal responsibilities that your spouse used to handle, you should discuss these with your spouse as early as possible following the diagnosis to ask all the questions you need to.

- ☐ In terms of finances, you need to know the following:

  - All accounts, checking or saving

  - All investments, such as all stock holdings

- All retirement accounts, such as a 401(k)s

- All debts, which is anything you are paying down, such as houses and cars

- All regular expenses, including when they need to be paid, on what schedule, and to whom

☐ If your loved one cannot provide the financial information you need, you'll have to do some digging:

- Find any statements you can, whether billing or account statements.

- Search on any computer your spouse may have used to manage your finances for emails indicating billing or account information.

- Look in any file cabinet (or similar storage place) you have for any documents related to your finances.

- Whatever you find, organize by type: bill for payment, checking account statement, savings account statement, 401(k) statement, etc.

- If you can't find the information you need but you have an institution you can contact, get in touch with the institution and explain your situation to them. They may be able to help you if they can verify your identity.

- It's possible that for any finance-related websites, your spouse kept a list of accounts and passwords somewhere, either in hard copy or in an electronic file. Look for anything like this, especially if your spouse ever mentioned something like it.

☐ If your loved one cannot provide the legal information you need:

- Contact your lawyer for more information.

- Look everywhere you can for any legal documents or other information you can find, whether in hard copy or electronic form.

- □ If you don't know what insurance your spouse may have:

  - ■ Look for anything that might verify this information in hard copy or electronic form.

  - ■ Look for insurance cards in your spouse's wallet or purse, nightstand, desk, or anywhere else they might be.

  - ■ If you can find the name of an insurance agent, contact the agent and explain your situation to find out all you can.

  - ■ Contact your spouse's current employer or last employer (if no longer working) to find out what they can tell you about any insurance your spouse might have had through them.

- □ Locate legal documents as soon as you can, and work with family to prepare and update essential legal documents such as a Durable Power of Attorney and your will. (For details on legal planning see *Advance Directives, Durable Power of Attorney, Wills, and Other Legal Considerations*).

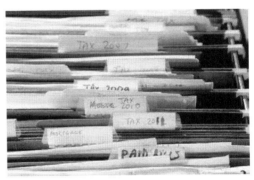

Credit: Image Steve Heap

- □ Organize financial accounts and documents as soon as possible, and work with family to understand insurance and your financial situation.

- □ You may feel overwhelmed by your new responsibilities. If in doubt, do not hesitate to turn to friends and family as well as financial and legal advisors and community resources that can help clarify your confusion.

Along with changing roles, dementia can cause changes in intimacy and sexuality in both a person with the disease and the caregiver. The person with the disease may be stressed by the changes in their memory and behaviors. Fear, worry, depression, anger, and low self-esteem are common. The person may become dependent and cling to you. They may not remember your life together and feelings for each other. They may even fall in love with someone else. You, the partner, may pull away in both an emotional and physical sense. You may be upset and frustrated by a sense of rejection as well as the strains of caregiving. You and your partner both have a need for intimacy, and it is likely that the form the intimacy takes will change as the disease progresses.

Checklist: Basics about changing physical and emotional intimacy

- ☐ To make your partner with dementia feel needed and loved, spend time with them. Tell your partner that you love them, you will keep them safe, and that others care about them.

- ☐ To address your own emotional needs, talk with a doctor, social worker, or clergy member about these changes. It helps to air out personal issues, though it may feel awkward to bring them up.

- ☐ Talk about your concerns in a support group.

- ☐ Think about the positive parts of your relationship with the person with dementia.

- ☐ Your partner may experience changes in sexuality, such as a seeming loss of interest in sex or hypersexuality, an extreme interest in sex.

- ☐ If your partner loses interest in sex or you don't feel comfortable engaging sexually with them, explore new ways of spending time together, focus on other ways to show affection, try nonsexual forms of touching, and explore other ways to meet your sexual needs.

- ☐ Hypersexuality, such as frequent masturbation or trying to seduce others, is a symptom of dementia. If your partner begins exhibiting signs of hypersexuality when you did not notice this before, this may be an effect of dementia, not necessarily a real desire for sex.

☐ To cope with hypersexuality, give the person attention and reassurance and show physical affection. If hypersexuality gets out of control, talk to a doctor.

If your spouse has been diagnosed with dementia, you will feel a range of emotions, including grief, as they gradually lose capabilities. You may experience grief as soon as your spouse is diagnosed, or it may become more prevalent as the condition progresses or when your spouse enters a long-term care facility. (For more information on living arrangements, see *Home Care, Long-term Care, Memory Care Units, and Other Living Arrangements*). You may experience "ambiguous loss," a form of grieving that takes place when your loved one's body remains but their memory is fading. No matter the form of your grief reaction, consider using these strategies to address your feelings.

Checklist: How to manage grief as a spouse's dementia progresses

☐ Find general advice on how to cope with grief.

☐ When your partner moves into a residential care facility, continue to be involved in caring for them.

☐ Teach the care staff about your partner's life history, preferences, and hobbies. You are likely to know your partner better than anyone, so this could greatly improve the quality of your loved one's care.

☐ If you feel you need time away from caregiving, take a break and allow long-term care staff to attend to your loved one's needs.

☐ When your partner passes away, allow yourself time and space to grieve. Don't cut ties with people in your life.

☐ Avoid making major decisions soon after your loved one passes away if you can.

☐ If it makes you comfortable, hold onto some of your loved one's treasured possessions. This may help you feel a sense of connection and ease the grieving process.

- [ ] Ask friends and family for support if you become overwhelmed by the grieving process or particular anniversaries or holidays.

- [ ] To readjust during and after bereavement, talk about your partner and your life together.

Adult Children

As the number of dementia diagnoses grows, so does the number of Americans charged with taking care of both their ailing parents and their own young families. People in the "sandwich generation" are required to constantly move between their roles as caretakers both of their parents and of their own children, a daunting task that

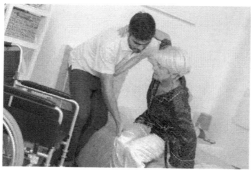

can take a major toll on a person's marriage, family, career, and health. Whether or not you have a family of your own—and whether or not you provide full-time care—adjusting to the role of caregiver to a parent with dementia can be a stressful and emotionally challenging task.

Credit: Image ALPA PROD

Checklist: Things to consider when taking care of your parent

- [ ] Try to accept your new role as caregiver as quickly as possible and prepare for the financial, legal, and medical steps that you will have to take as caregiver over the course of your parent's illness.

- [ ] Your parent might live a long time after diagnosis. Many people with dementia live ten or more years after the initial diagnosis.

- [ ] The demands on you as a caregiver will grow larger over time. In the early stages, a primary caregiver may spend around ten hours every week providing care, but in the latter stages that number can rise to around 40 hours or more.

- The responsibilities of caregiving will affect your career, family, and finances, particularly if you are a full-time caregiver.

- Reach out to the rest of your family and your close friends when you need help coping with the duties of caregiving. Getting rest is essential to maintaining your relationship with your parent and your ability to provide high-quality care.

- Accept that your relationship with your parent is changing and that it will continue to evolve as your parent loses their memory capabilities. Acknowledge these changes and share your thoughts and feelings with loved ones.

- Focus on the quality of your relationship with your parent by taking time to engage in fun activities with them. As much as possible, do things that you used to do together, go outside for a walk, or spend time with family.

- If you are a caregiver with children of your own, explain the situation to your children in an age-appropriate manner. With younger children, explain to them that dementia is not contagious and that they did not cause it. Keep them updated on the status of your parent and let them know about your caregiving responsibilities.

- Involve your own children in caregiving if possible, and meet as a family to talk about the situation.

- To maintain your relationship with your own immediate family, spend time with your children without your parent. It is good for everyone if you disengage periodically from caregiving and spend time in a more relaxed context.

When you and your family take on caregiving responsibilities as a team, you have the ability to lessen the stress of caregiving for everyone. With more people around to share the work of caregiving, the burden is lighter for all. However, with more people making decisions about your loved one's care, there is a greater chance for miscommunication, disagreement, and even mistrust to develop, all of which can damage your relationships as well as impede quality caregiving. (Also see the section on the causes of and strategies for resolving conflict in *Advance Directives, Durable Power of Attorney, Wills, and Other Legal Considerations.*) Following the suggestions in the checklist below will help you maintain emotionally healthy relationships with family members.

Checklist: Things to consider when sharing responsibility with family members

- ☐ Acknowledge that not every family member will agree about the ways in which care should be given.

- ☐ Differences of opinion will inevitably crop up in complicated legal, financial, and medical situations, and accepting these disagreements is essential to providing high-quality care. (For details on legal planning see *Advance Directives, Durable Power of Attorney, Wills, and Other Legal Considerations*).

- ☐ In family crises, adult children frequently revert to their old family roles. For example, the oldest child might be expected to make all the hard decisions. Gender stereotyping can also play a role; women may be expected to provide more care than male siblings.

- ☐ Recognize that you all benefit from working together. The burden of providing full-time care alone is exhausting and sometimes downright impossible, so try to work through your differences for the good of your loved one.

- ☐ Divide labor so that everyone provides care suited to their abilities, strengths, and life situation. A daughter who lives far away might handle financial duties, while sons who live closer to their parent with dementia might assist with day-to-day caregiving.

- ☐ Share important information so that everyone can make reasonable decisions and so that mistrust does not develop.

- ☐ Make sure that all relevant family members are copied on relevant communications and that everyone who needs them has access to essential documents.

- ☐ Check in with one another regularly so that the whole family is aware of your loved one's condition. Try to avoid communicating only with the family members to whom you feel closest; include other family members too.

☐ At big decision and crisis points, schedule family meetings or teleconferences so that everyone's voice can be heard.

☐ Do not criticize your family members' caregiving efforts. Even if you feel that they are doing a subpar job or that the burden is falling on you, frame your criticism positively.

☐ Avoid making promises you cannot keep, such as a promise not to put a loved one into full-time residential care. Denial and fear of breaking promises are at the root of much guilt and disagreement.

☐ When appropriate, bring in outside help, such as an in-home care provider or a geriatric care manager. Having a neutral third party around can provide a mediator for families while they are making tough decisions.

Emotional Considerations for Non-Caregiver Family and Friends

If you are a family member or a friend of an individual who has been diagnosed with dementia, you may have sensed that something has been wrong with your loved one for a while. When you hear about their diagnosis, you may be confused, saddened, and unsure of how to relate to the person with the disease. There is no single

correct way to adjust when someone in your life has dementia, but you owe it to yourself and them to try to understand the changes the disease brings and how you can continue to have a positive relationship with the person.

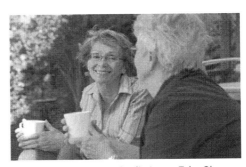

Credit: Image Tyler Olsen

Checklist: Things to consider when accepting and understanding the changes associated with dementia

- ☐ Research dementia to discover what is realistic to expect that your loved one can and cannot do and the likely course of their disease.

- ☐ Talk to primary caregivers to try to understand your loved one's capabilities and the ways in which they are changing.

- ☐ If the person seemingly does not remember you, make eye contact and introduce yourself, giving them a cue to help them remember you. Speak to the person naturally regardless of whether they seem to remember you.

- ☐ Avoid correcting the person with dementia if they make a mistake or forget something. Respond to the feelings the person expresses or talk about something different.

- ☐ In the early stages of dementia, plan fun activities with the person, such as going to family reunions or visiting old friends. A photo album or other activity can help if the person is bored or confused and needs to be distracted.

- ☐ Visit at times of the day when the person with dementia is likely to be at their best.

- ☐ Be calm and quiet. Don't use a loud voice or talk to the person as if they were a child.

- ☐ Respect the person's personal space and don't get too close.

- ☐ Do not take it personally if the person does not recognize you, is unkind, or gets angry. They are likely acting out of confusion.

When a family member has dementia, it affects everyone in the family, including children and grandchildren. It is important to talk to them about what is happening. How much and what kind of information you share depends on the child's age and relationship to the person with dementia.

☐ Answer children's questions simply and honestly. For example, you might tell a young child, "Grandma has an illness that makes it hard for her to remember things."

☐ Help them understand that their feelings of sadness and anger are normal.

☐ Comfort them. Tell them no one caused the disease.

☐ Talk with kids about their concerns and feelings. Some may not talk about their negative feelings, but you may see changes in how they act.

☐ Note problems at school because they may indicate an expression of emotional distress. A school counselor or social worker can help your child understand what is happening and how to cope.

☐ For both the person with dementia and the child or teenager, spending time together is important. You may be able to set up activities to facilitate this such as doing arts and crafts, playing music, looking through photo albums, and reading stories out loud.

☐ A teenager might find it hard to accept how the person with dementia has changed. They may find the changes upsetting or embarrassing to be around. Even as you encourage your teen to spend time with the person with dementia, do not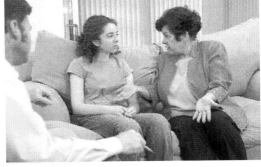

Credit: Image Lisa F. Young

force them to spend time with the person.

☐ If the child or teenager lives in the same house as the person with dementia, do not expect them to look after the person with dementia unless they have said they want to and you have determined that they can handle the responsibility.

- ☐ Ensure that children and teens in close proximity with your loved one have time for their own interests and needs.

- ☐ Make sure that you spend time with children and teens so that they don't feel that all your attention is on the person with dementia.

- ☐ Be honest about your feelings when you talk with kids but don't overwhelm them.

When your family member or friend is diagnosed with dementia and you are not a primary caregiver, you might have mixed feelings about your role. You might feel excluded from providing care for the person when you want to help, or you may simply not know what help is needed or wanted. The most important thing you can do for your loved one is to remain by their side and to provide relief to the family and primary caregivers when they need it.

Checklist: Emotional considerations for non-caregiver family and friends

- ☐ Educate yourself about dementia to get rid of any preconceptions you might have about the disease. Misconceptions can compromise your relationship with the person with dementia.

- ☐ Do not think too hard about what you will talk about when visiting the person. Talk in the same way you always have, and adjust your tone or subject matter as appropriate to the person's condition.

- ☐ If you cannot be physically present for the person, send a note or a card. Make sure the person knows you care.

- ☐ Don't allow the person's status as someone with dementia to define the whole way that you see them. Remember your personal history with the person.

- ☐ When visiting the person with dementia, look friendly, make eye contact, and offer some form of greeting.

- [ ] Be physically at the person's level to engage them directly. Discuss your history together rather than recent details or events. Don't berate the person if they don't remember something correctly.

- [ ] Speak with a level tone, staying positive and allowing frequent pauses for the person to contribute.

- [ ] Engage in an activity with the person rather than just talking. Bring a prompt such as old pictures or music that the person enjoys.

- [ ] Make the person aware of what you intend to do before you act, especially if it involves touching them.

- [ ] Offer to provide respite care to give the caregiver time for themselves. Don't just say "Let me know if you need anything." Instead, plan a specific time that you are available to provide respite care so the caregiver can have time away. This will provide incredible emotional support to the caregiver, and it will let the person with dementia know that you care.

Coping with the Behavioral Changes of Dementia

For both dementia caregivers and non-caregivers, knowing how to contend with the emotional symptoms of the condition is important for minimizing stress and optimizing care for the person with dementia. The memory loss associated with dementia gives rise to a wide range of seemingly unrelated and sometimes unpredictable emotional effects, such as agitation and aggression, delusions and hallucinations, personality changes, confusion at sundown, and changes in communication skills. Realize that when your loved one shows these behaviors, it is the disease talking.

As dementia progresses, if your loved one becomes agitated or aggressive, look for a cause. Most of the time, agitation and aggression happen for a reason. If you can identify and address the cause, the behavior may stop. For example, the person may be experiencing pain, depression, stress, too little rest or sleep, or loneliness. Look for early signs of agitation or aggression. If you see the signs, you can deal with the causes before problem behaviors start. Try not to ignore the problem. Doing nothing can make things worse and may result in more stress and agitation for you and your loved one.

Checklist: How to cope with agitation and aggression

- ☐ Reassure the person. Speak calmly. Listen to their concerns and frustrations. Try to show that you understand if the person is angry or fearful.

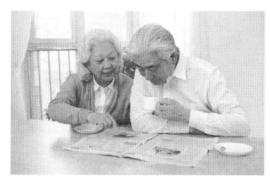
Credit: Image Eastfenceimage

- ☐ Allow the person to keep as much control in their life as possible.

- ☐ Try to keep a routine, such as bathing, dressing, and eating at the same time each day.

- ☐ Build quiet times into the day along with activities.

- ☐ Keep well-loved objects and photographs around the house to help the person feel more secure.

- ☐ Try gentle touching, soothing music, reading, or walks.

- ☐ Reduce noise, clutter, or the number of people in the room.

- ☐ Try to distract the person with a favorite snack, object, or activity.

- ☐ Limit the amount of caffeine, sugar, and "junk food" the person drinks and eats.

- ☐ Slow down and try to relax if you think your own worries may be affecting the person with dementia.

- ☐ Try to find a way to take a break from caregiving.

☐ When the person is aggressive, protect yourself and others. If you have to, stay at a safe distance from the person until the behavior stops. Also try to protect the person from hurting themselves.

As dementia progresses, the person with the disease may have hallucinations, delusions, or paranoia. During a hallucination, the person sees, hears, smells, tastes, or feels something that isn't there. They also may have delusions, or false beliefs, that the person thinks are real. Paranoia is a type of delusion in which a person may believe—without a good reason—that others are mean, lying, unfair, or out to get them. They may become suspicious, fearful, or jealous of people. Paranoia may be the person's way of expressing loss. The person may blame or accuse others because no other explanation seems to make sense.

Checklist: How to cope with delusions and hallucinations

☐ Discuss with the doctor any illnesses the person with dementia has and medicine they are taking. Sometimes an illness or medicine may cause hallucinations or delusions.

☐ Try not to argue with the person about what they see or hear. To them, the hallucination is real. Comfort the person if they are afraid.

☐ Distract the person. Sometimes moving to another room or going outside for a walk helps.

☐ Turn off the TV when violent or upsetting programs are on. Someone with dementia may think these events are happening in the room.

☐ Make sure the person is safe and can't reach anything that could be used to hurt anyone or themselves.

☐ Try not to react if the person blames you for something.

☐ Don't argue with the person.

☐ Let the person know that they are safe.

☐ Use gentle touching or hugging to show you care.

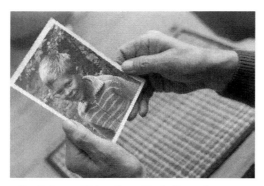

☐ Search for things to distract the person, then talk about what you found. For example, talk about a photograph or keepsake.

☐ Explain to others that the person is acting this way because they have dementia.

☐ Keep in mind that someone with dementia may have a good reason for acting a certain way. They may not be paranoid. There are people who take advantage of weak and elderly people. Find out if someone is trying to abuse or steal from your loved one.

The progression of dementia affects not only memory but also how a person acts. These checklists provide suggestions that may help you understand and cope with changes in personality and behavior in a person with dementia.

Checklist: Common personality and behavior changes

☐ Getting easily upset

☐ Acting depressed

☐ Hiding things

☐ Wandering

☐ Showing unusual sexual behavior

☐ Hitting caregivers

☐ No longer caring about how they look

☐ No longer bathing

☐ Wanting to wear the same clothes every day

Checklist: How to cope with personality and behavior changes

☐ Keep things simple. Ask or say one thing at a time.

☐ Have a daily routine so that the person knows when certain things will happen.

☐ Reassure the person that they are safe and you are there to help.

☐ Focus on their feelings rather than words. For example, say, "You seem worried."

☐ Don't argue or try to reason with the person.

☐ Try not to show your frustration or anger. If you get upset, take deep breaths and count to 10. If it's safe, leave the room for a few minutes.

☐ Use humor when you can.

☐ If your loved one paces, give them a safe place to walk.

☐ Try using music, singing, or dancing to distract the person. Remember to set the stage a bit. Just putting on music or beginning to sing or dance might not help. Say, "Why don't we take a break and listen to some music," and then watch and build on any positive reaction you see.

☐ Ask for help. For instance, say, "Let's set the table" or "I need help folding the clothes."

☐ Talk with the person's doctor about problems such as hitting, biting, depression, or hallucinations. Medications are available to treat some behavioral symptoms.

Late afternoon and early evening can be difficult for some people with dementia. They may experience sundowning—restlessness, agitation, irritability, or confusion that can begin or worsen as daylight begins to fade—often just when tired caregivers need a break. Sundowning can continue into the night, making it hard for people with dementia to fall asleep and stay in bed. As a result, they and their caregivers may have trouble getting enough sleep and functioning well during the day. The causes of sundowning are not well understood. One possibility is that dementia can lead to brain changes that affect a person's sleep-wake cycle. This may result in agitation and other sundowning behaviors. Other possible causes of sundowning include being overly tired, unmet needs such as hunger or thirst, depression, pain, and boredom.

Checklist: How to cope with sundowning

- ☐ Look for signs of sundowning in the late afternoon and early evening. These signs may include increased confusion or anxiety and behaviors such as pacing, wandering, or yelling.

- ☐ If you can, try to find the cause of your loved one's behavior. If they become agitated, listen calmly to their concerns and frustrations. Try to reassure the person that everything is OK and distract them from stressful or upsetting events.

- ☐ Reduce noise, clutter, or the number of people in the room.

- ☐ Try to distract the person with a favorite snack, object, or activity. For example, offer a drink, suggest a simple task such as folding towels, or turn on a familiar TV show (but not shows that might be upsetting).

- ☐ Make early evening a quiet time of day. You might play soothing music, read, or go for a walk. You could also have a family member or friend call during this time.

- ☐ Close the curtains or blinds at dusk to minimize shadows and the confusion they may cause. Turn on lights to help minimize shadows.

- ☐ Reduce the person's tiredness by going outside or at least sitting by the window. Exposure to bright light can help reset the person's body clock.

- ☐ Help the person get physical activity or exercise each day. If this makes the person tired, have them take a nap, but keep naps short and not too late in the day to ensure the person gets enough rest at night.

- ☐ Avoid serving coffee, cola, or other drinks with caffeine late in the day.

- [ ] Avoid serving alcoholic drinks. They may add to confusion and anxiety.

- [ ] Avoid planning too many activities during the day. A full schedule can be tiring.

- [ ] If sundowning continues to be a problem, seek medical advice. A medical exam may identify the cause of sundowning, such as pain, a sleep disorder or other illness, or a medication side effect.

- [ ] If medication is prescribed to help the person relax and sleep better at night, be sure to find out about possible side effects. Some medications can increase the chances of dizziness, falls, and confusion. Doctors recommend using them only for short periods of time.

Behavioral changes involving communication are among the most difficult to deal with because they cut you off from what the person is thinking and feeling. Communication is hard for people with dementia because they have trouble remembering things. They may struggle to find words or forget what they want to say. You may feel impatient and wish they could just say what they want, but they can't.

The person with dementia may have problems with finding the right word, losing their train of thought when speaking, understanding what words mean, or paying attention during long conversations. Your loved one may also have trouble remembering the steps in common activities; blocking out background noises from the radio, TV, or conversations; and being very sensitive to touch and to the tone and loudness of voices.

Checklist: How to cope with changes in communication skills

- [ ] Make eye contact and call the person by name.

- [ ] Be aware of your tone, how loud your voice is, how you look at your loved one, and your body language.

- [ ] Encourage a two-way conversation for as long as possible.

- [ ] Use other methods besides speaking, such as gentle touching.

- ☐ Try distracting the person if communication creates problems.

- ☐ Use a warm, loving, matter-of-fact manner.

- ☐ Hold your loved one's hand while you talk.

- ☐ Be open to your loved one's concerns, even if they are hard to understand.

- ☐ Let them make some decisions and stay involved.

- ☐ Be patient with angry outbursts. Remember, it's the illness "talking."

- ☐ Offer simple, step-by-step instructions.

- ☐ Repeat instructions and allow more time for a response. Try not to interrupt.

- ☐ Don't talk about your loved one as if they aren't there.

- ☐ Don't talk to the person using "baby talk" or a "baby voice."

- ☐ Ask questions that require a yes or no answer. For example, you could say, "Are you tired?" instead of "How do you feel?"

- ☐ Limit the number of choices. For example, you could say, "Would you like a hamburger or chicken for dinner?" instead of "What would you like for dinner?"

- ☐ Use different words if your loved one doesn't understand the first time. For example, if you ask the person whether they are hungry and you don't get a response, you could say, "Dinner is ready now. Let's eat."

- ☐ Try not to say, "Don't you remember?" or "I told you."

- ☐ If you become frustrated, take some time out for yourself.

Receiving Emotional Support

The emotional burden of dementia can be a lot for one family to handle, but community resources offer a respite from the day-to-day anxiety of caring for a loved one with the disease. Government, community, and religious organizations all offer assistance, from daycare services to transportation resources, that can ease the emotional strain on both caregiver and loved one. See the Resources for more information on community and faith-based support.

Checklist: Basics about community and faith-based support

☐ Adult day services can provide social and recreational activities as well as meals. Some provide nursing care, treatment plans, transportation services, and caregiver support groups.

☐ Most adult day services offer daytime weekday services, with a few providing night and weekend hours. These services offer people with dementia additional care, and they offer caregivers respite time.

☐ Assisted living and residential care services provide more comprehensive care for people with dementia. These services offer 24/7 monthly care. (For more information on living arrangements, see *Home Care, Long-term Care, Memory Care Units, and Other Living Arrangements.*)

☐ Government aging resources include health centers, Agencies on Aging, family support divisions of local governments, and ombudsman programs, which investigate abuse and neglect claims against public authorities.

☐ Home-delivered meals programs can take the stress out of preparing food for a loved one.

☐ In-home agencies provide care resources in your or your loved one's own home. Using an in-home care agency can reduce the amount of time

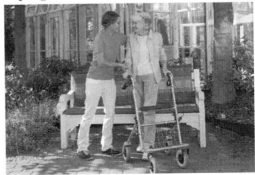

Credit: Image belushi

you spend on caregiving each day as well as reduce the stress of providing services you do not feel qualified for.

- ☐ Dementia-related driving resources include classes administered by local entities as well as assessments issued by the state DMV.

- ☐ Transportation resources include private shuttle services and bus services offered by local community centers and senior citizens' clubs.

- ☐ Local classes for people with dementia are frequently administered by medical practitioners and the Alzheimer's Association and provide support group, education, and brain fitness services.

Support groups and formal counseling services can directly address emotional strain by placing your experience in context and resolving long-standing tensions.

Checklist: Basics about support groups

- ☐ Support groups offer a space to converse with other people impacted by dementia. In a support group, you can share your experience and learn from others in similar situations.

- ☐ Many support groups meet monthly and many are free. Some even offer transportation and care services.

- ☐ The Alzheimer's Association provides a comprehensive listing of available support groups on its website. See the Resources for more information.

- ☐ Message boards offer many of the same advantages as local support groups but without the need for physical meetings. Sign into an online message board to share stories, discuss common experiences, and seek caregiving advice. See the Resources for more information.

- ☐ If you're in need of instant advice on a caregiving matter, an Alzheimer's disease helpline can provide reliable information in a pinch. The Alzheimer's Association runs a toll-free 24/7 line at 1-800-272-3900.

- [ ] Support groups, message boards, and helplines can provide support and guidance concerning the basics of dementia, medications and treatment, general information about aging, caregiving skills, and legal concerns.

Checklist: Basics about counseling and therapy

- [ ] The emotional impacts of caring for someone with dementia can be significant due to the long-term nature of the disease. If you or your loved one feels chronically or overwhelmingly anxious or depressed about dementia, consider seeking counseling or therapy.

- [ ] Counseling is typically a relatively short-term process that focuses on addressing specific issues such as stress or anger through problem-solving techniques.

- [ ] Therapy is generally a longer-term process that seeks to uncover someone's unconscious thinking patterns and teach more positive ways of thinking.

- [ ] Many people hesitate to seek mental health services because they feel embarrassed to admit weakness. Don't hesitate to seek out these services if you need help. There's no shame in admitting that you need assistance when you are responsible for the overwhelming task of caring for someone with dementia.

- [ ] To get in touch with a therapist who can help you or a loved one cope with the effects of dementia, ask for a referral from your primary care physician or seek out a social worker, family therapist, psychologist, or psychiatrist whose practice is suited to your particular needs.

- [ ] The mental health provider you meet with will conduct an initial interview, asking you about your symptoms, your medical history, and why you are seeking counseling.

- [ ] Based on this survey, the provider will discuss counseling options, including where the counseling will take place, who will be involved, and how long and how often you should go to counseling.

Checklist: Types of counseling for dementia

☐ Crisis intervention counseling provides an immediate solution in times of dire emotional need. Alzheimer's disease helplines and suicide prevention hotlines frequently provide these services.

☐ Individual counseling provides one-on-one conversation for someone struggling with the effects of dementia. Individual counseling works best when problems stem from one's own thinking patterns and behaviors, manifested as grief, anxiety, and depression.

☐ Family therapy provides a space for family members to directly address interpersonal conflicts originating from a dementia diagnosis. Participants can air their grievances in a productive manner as well as realize that they are not isolated individuals in addressing dementia.

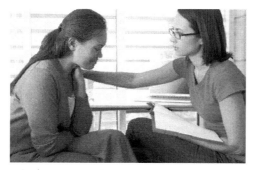
Credit: Image Monkey Business Images

☐ Long-term residential treatment is a therapy option in which the patient reduces involvement in other areas of their life to focus on getting better. In long-term residential therapy, counseling and group therapy work hand in hand to help someone understand their own thought processes.

☐ Mental health self-help, support groups, and co-counseling provide formal structures for people to share their problems and understand possible solutions. Many of these groups are conducted with the help of a licensed therapist or counselor.

Conclusion

The emotional fallout of a dementia diagnosis in the family affects everyone differently. The person with dementia must come to terms with their diagnosis and do what they can to live a fulfilling life within the limitations imposed by the condition. Their caregivers must reckon with the grief of a loved one being diagnosed with a terminal illness while simultaneously trying to reduce the intense stress of caregiving. In addition, other family members and friends must process their own feelings about the diagnosis while helping where they can and providing emotional support to those closest to the disease.

Remember that as someone affected by dementia, you can reduce emotional strain in two ways: by lessening the stress of caregiving and by lessening the effects of that stress. To reduce the stress on your family, share the load of caregiving or take on some of the burden. To reduce the effects of stress, look out for your physical, emotional, and social health. See a doctor regularly, and perhaps most importantly, keep in touch with loved ones. Cultivating a healthy social network can reduce the emotional struggle of dementia and bring family and friends closer together.

About the Authors

Laura Town

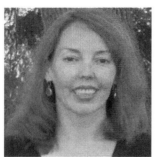

Laura Town has authored numerous publications of special interest to the aging population. She has expertise in the field of finance as a co-author on *Finance: Foundations of Financial Institutions and Management* published by John Wiley and Sons, and she has contributed to several online nursing courses and texts. She has also written for the American Medical Writers Association, and her work has been published by the American Society of Journalists and Authors. As an editor, Laura has worked with Pearson Education, Prentice Hall, McGraw-Hill Higher Education, John Wiley and Sons, and the University of Pennsylvania to create both on-ground and online courses and texts. She is the past president of the Indiana chapter of the American Medical Writers Association.

Karen Hoffman

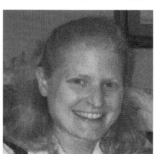

Karen (Kassel) Hoffman received her Ph.D. in Pharmacology from the Department of Pharmacology and Experimental Neurosciences at the University of Nebraska Medical Center in Omaha, NE, where she was the recipient of an American Heart Association fellowship and several regional and national awards for her research on G protein-coupled receptor signaling in airways. She then pursued post-doctoral research projects at the University of North Carolina-Chapel Hill and the University of Kansas Medical Center, again receiving fellowships from the PhRMA Foundation and the American Heart Association, respectively. She has published research in the *American Journal of Pathology*, *Journal of Biological Chemistry*, and *Journal of*

Pharmacology and Experimental Therapeutics. In 2012, Karen joined the editorial staff at WilliamsTown Communications, an editing firm that specializes in educational products for undergraduate- and graduate-level students. At WTC, Karen specializes in producing educational products related to the sciences and healthcare. In addition, Karen is board-certified for editing life sciences (BELS-certified).

A Note from the Authors

Thank you for purchasing our book! Worldwide, over forty million people suffer from Alzheimer's disease, and that number is expected to increase significantly within the next fifteen years. In the United States, over five million people have the disease, and that is expected to triple by the year 2050.

Despite these large numbers, you may feel alone. I (Laura) know that when I started caring for my father, who had early-onset Alzheimer's disease, I felt alone. Although my father has passed away, I am haunted by what he suffered and how difficult it was to care for him. However, now I know that there are people, resources, and organizations that can help others going through this same struggle.

We recognize that caregivers have emotional, physical, and financial challenges. We hope that the information in the *Alzheimer's Roadmap* series will ease some of your stress. The information included in this book can help you manage your stress and emotions related to your loved one's diagnosis. In addition, we have included resources at the end of this book to provide additional information to help you through this process.

If you have any questions for us, feel free to post them on Laura Town's Amazon Author Central page or reach out to the authors via twitter: @laurawtown. We would appreciate it if you would take the time to review our book on Amazon, as our book's visibility on Amazon depends on reviews.

More Titles from Laura Town and Karen Hoffman

Alzheimer's Roadmap series:

Long-Term Care Insurance, Power of Attorney, Wealth Management, and Other First Steps

Dementia, Alzheimer's Disease Stages, Treatments, and Other Medical Considerations

Advance Directives, Durable Power of Attorney, Wills, and Other Legal Considerations

Paying for Healthcare and Other Financial Considerations

Home Safety Checklist Guide and Caregiver Resources for Medication Safety, Driving, and Wandering

Home Care, Long-term Care, Memory Care Units, and Other Living Arrangements

Enhancing the Activities of Daily Living

Nutrition for Brain Health: Fighting Dementia

Caregiver Resources: From Independence to a Memory Care Unit

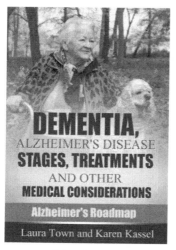

A guide to Alzheimer's disease, how it progresses, and how to treat it

Dementia, Alzheimer's Disease Stages, Treatments, and Other Medical Considerations provides answers to the following questions and more:

- **What is Alzheimer's disease?** This book describes what Alzheimer's disease is, including its characteristics, warning signs, and risk factors.
- **What can my loved one with Alzheimer's disease expect?** Read detailed descriptions of the general stages of Alzheimer's disease, including what patients and caregivers can expect to see at each stage as the disease progresses.
- **What treatments are available?** A survey of prescription medications introduces you to the treatments available to help patients with Alzheimer's disease cope with the progression of the disease. Also find out which drugs to avoid. An additional review of alternative treatments assesses the efficacy and veracity of some of these treatments.

> "Best resource I have found for explaining in terms I can understand about what my husband is experiencing and will be going through."
>
> Kindle Customer

- **What about clinical trials?** Clinical trials are important to finding a cure for Alzheimer's disease, but this book describes the precautions your loved one to consider before choosing to participate in them.
- **Is there audio for this book?** Yes, you can find the audiobook here: **https://amzn.to/2TjQT0W**

Simple dietary changes can improve cognition and decrease dementia risk and progression

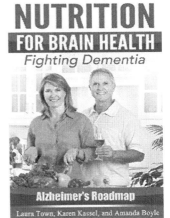

Nutrition for Brain Health: Fighting Dementia provides answers to the following questions and more:

- **How can what I eat affect my brain health?** Discover how to lower you risk factors for dementia by decreasing your intake of saturated fats and cholesterol, balancing your diet, and controlling the calories you consume.
- **Do I need to exercise?** Explore the various ways that everyday activities can double as brain-enhancing exercise and improve your total health as well.
- **Does what I drink matter?** Find out how some things you may drink, such as coffee, tea, or red wine, can actually be beneficial for brain health in moderation.
- **How do I get the vitamins I need?** Know what dietary and lifestyle choices can increase your intake of essential vitamins such as vitamins C and B_{12}.
- **How do I know what specific foods are good for me?** This book defines the elements of a healthy, balanced diet and then goes beyond that to identify the specific foods that will give you the nutrients you need to extend and improve cognitive function.
- **Is there an electronic version of this book?** Yes, and it's free!
- **Is there an audio version of this book?** Yes, there is. You can find it at: https://adbl.co/2Vwbe0d

Resources

Information Resources:

Alzheimer's Association
225 N. Michigan Ave., Fl. 17
Chicago, IL 60601-7633
Phone: 800-272-3900
Fax: 866-699-1246
Email: info@alz.org
Website: http://www.alz.org
Identify local resources with the "In My Community" feature:
http://www.alz.org/apps/findus.asp

Alzheimer's Foundation of America
322 Eighth Ave., 7th fl.
New York, NY 10001
Phone: 866-232-8484
Fax: 646-638-1546
Website: www.alzfdn.org

American Association of Retired Persons
Website: http://aarp.org

Fisher's Center for Alzheimer's Research Foundation
199 Water Street, 23rd Floor
New York, NY 10038
Phone: 1-800-259-4636
Fax: 1-212-915-1319
Email: info@alzinfo.org
Website: http://www.alzinfo.org

Support Groups:
Alzheimer's Association Support Group Directory and Message Boards
Website:
http://www.alz.org/apps/we_can_help/support_groups.asp

Alzheimer's Disease Centers
Phone: 1-800-438-4380
Website: http://www.nia.nih.gov/alzheimers/alzheimers-disease-research-centers

Alzheimer's Foundation of America
Phone: 1-866-232-8484
Website: http://www.alzfdn.org/

Caring.com Online Support Groups
Website: https://www.caring.com/support-groups

NIH Alzheimer's Disease Education and Referral (ADEAR) Center
Phone: 1-800-438-4380
Website: http://www.nia.nih.gov/alzheimers

Family Caregiver Alliance
Phone: 1-800-445-8106
Website: https://caregiver.org/

Caregiver Respite Services:
Alzheimer's Association
Phone: 1.800.272.3900
Website:
http://www.alz.org/national/documents/brochure_respitecareguide.pdf

Arch National Respite Network and Resource Center
Website: http://archrespite.org/respitelocator

Eldercare Locator
Phone: 1-800-677-1116.
Website:
http://www.eldercare.gov/Eldercare.NET/Public/Index.aspx

Mental Health Directories:
GoodTherapy

Website: http://www.goodtherapy.org/

Psychology Today's Therapy Directory
Website: https://therapists.psychologytoday.com/rms/

Therapist Referral Network
Phone: 1-800-843-7274
Phone: 1-858-481-1515

MedicarePhysican Compare
Locate providers who accept Medicare.
Website: http://www.medicare.gov/physiciancompare/

National Association of Medicaid Directors
Locate providers who accept Medicaid.
Website: http://medicaiddirectors.org/

Physician Directories:
WebMD Physician Directory
Website: http://doctor.webmd.com/

American Medical Association DoctorFinder
Website: https://apps.ama-assn.org/doctorfinder/recaptcha.jsp

MedicarePhysican Compare
Locate providers who accept Medicare.
Website: http://www.medicare.gov/physiciancompare/

National Association of Medicaid Directors
Locate providers who accept Medicaid.
Website: http://medicaiddirectors.org/

Elder Abuse Reporting and Prevention:
National Center on Elder Abuse State Resources
Website:
http://ncea.aoa.gov/Stop_Abuse/Get_Help/State/index.aspx

Eldercare Locator

Phone: 1-800-677-1116
Website:
http://www.eldercare.gov/Eldercare.NET/Public/Index.aspx

<u>The National Consumer Voice for Quality Long-Term Care</u>
Locate an ombudsman for nursing home abuse.
Website: http://theconsumervoice.org/get_help

Reference List

AgingCare.com. (2019). Left unchecked, caregiver burnout can lead to abuse and violence. Retrieved from http://www.agingcare.com/Articles/caregivers-kill-parents-commit-suicide-150336.htm.

Akers, J. 4 powerful tips to reduce resentment and feel happier. *tiny buddha*. Retrieved from https://tinybuddha.com/blog/4-powerful-tips-to-reduce-resentment-and-feel-happier/.

AlzheimerSociety Canada. (2015). Quality of life. Retrieved from http://www.alzheimer.ca/en/Living-with-dementia/Caring-for-someone/Quality-of-life.

Alzheimer's Association. (2019). Retrieved from http://www.alz.org/.

Alzheimer's Association. (2019). 10 early signs and symptoms of Alzheimer's. Retrieved from https://www.alz.org/alzheimers-dementia/10_signs.

Alzheimer's Society. (2017). Grief, loss, and bereavement. Retrieved from http://alzheimers.org.uk/factsheet/507.

American Association of Retired Persons. (2015). Caregiving in the U.S. Retrieved from https://www.caregiving.org/wp-content/uploads/2015/05/2015_CaregivingintheUS_Executive-Summary-June-4_WEB.pdf.

American Foundation for Suicide Prevention. (2019). Risk factors and warning signs. Retrieved from https://afsp.org/about-suicide/risk-factors-and-warning-signs/.

Anxiety.org. (2017). How deep breathing can treat and reduce anxiety. Retrieved from https://www.anxiety.org/autogenic-relaxation.

BrightFocus Foundation. (2019). Managing Stress: Caring for the caregiver. Retrieved from https://www.brightfocus.org/alzheimers/news/managing-stress-caring-caregiver.

Caring.com. (2019). How to avoid strained sibling relationship relationships when a parent has Alzheimer's. *DailyCaring*. Retrieved from https://www.caring.com/articles/sibling-relationships-strained.

Caring Bridge (2019). Retrieved from https://www.caringbridge.org/.

Chand, S. (2018). Reducing suicide risk. Anxiety and Depression Association of America. Retrieved from https://adaa.org/learn-from-us/from-the-experts/blog-posts/consumer/reducing-suicide-risk.

Cleveland Clinic. (2019). Guided imagery. Retrieved from https://my.clevelandclinic.org/departments/wellness/integrative/treatments-services/guided-imagery#what-we-treat-tab.

Fontana, J. (2018). 6 ways to nurture your emotional health. *Headway*. Retrieved from https://headway.ginger.io/6-ways-to-nurture-your-emotional-health-dfd3194d9a3c.

Get Sleep. (2008). Address your sleep issues. Retrieved from http://healthysleep.med.harvard.edu/need-sleep/what-can-you-do/sleep-address-issues.

Harvard Health Publishing. (2016). Six relaxation techniques to reduce stress. Retrieved from https://www.health.harvard.edu/mind-and-mood/six-relaxation-techniques-to-reduce-stress.

Helpguide.org. (2019). Retrieved from http://www.helpguide.org/.

Holland, E. (2007). Chronic stress can steal years from caregivers' lifetimes. *OSU Research News*. Retrieved from https://news.osu.edu/chronic-stress-can-steal-years-from-caregivers-lifetimes---091807/.

Larkin, C. B. (2016). Denial is dangerous in dementia care. *Alzheimer's Reading Room*. Retrieved from http://www.alzheimersreadingroom.com/2010/04/denial-is-dangerous.html.

Mager, D. (2017). 8 strategies to work through anger and resentment. *Psychology Today*. Retrieved from https://www.psychologytoday.com/us/blog/some-assembly-required/201701/8-strategies-work-through-anger-and-resentment.

Marley, M. (2013). 10 tips for visiting a friend with Alzheimer's. *The Huffington Post*. Retrieved from http://www.huffingtonpost.com/marie-marley/10-tips-for-visiting-a-friend-with-alzheimers_b_4052740.html.

Mayo Clinic. (2019). Aerobic exercise. Retrieved from https://www.mayoclinic.org/healthy-lifestyle/fitness/basics/aerobic-exercise/hlv-20049447.

Mayo Clinic. (2019). Alzheimer's stages: How the disease progresses. Retrieved from https://www.mayoclinic.org/diseases-conditions/alzheimers-disease/in-depth/alzheimers-stages/art-20048448.

Mayo Clinic. (2019). Anxiety disorders. Retrieved from https://www.mayoclinic.org/diseases-conditions/anxiety/symptoms-causes/syc-20350961.

Mayo Clinic. (2019). Can music help someone with Alzheimer's? Retrieved from https://www.mayoclinic.org/diseases-conditions/alzheimers-disease/expert-answers/music-and-alzheimers/faq-20058173.

Mayo Clinic. (2019). Complicated grief. Retrieved from https://www.mayoclinic.org/diseases-conditions/complicated-grief/symptoms-causes/syc-20360374.

Mayo Clinic. (2019). Depression (major depressive disorder). Retrieved from https://www.mayoclinic.org/diseases-conditions/depression/symptoms-causes/syc-20356007.

Mayo Clinic. (2017). Relaxation techniques: Try these steps to reduce stress. Retrieved from https://www.mayoclinic.org/healthy-lifestyle/stress-management/in-depth/relaxation-technique/art-20045368.

MedlinePlus. (2019). Grief. Retrieved from http://www.nlm.nih.gov/medlineplus/ency/article/001530.htm.

MentalHelp.net. (2019). Treatment: When to seek professional help and where to find help for major depression. Retrieved from https://www.mentalhelp.net/depression/when-to-seek-professional-help/.

National Institute on Aging. (n.d.). Alzheimer's caregiving. Retrieved from https://www.nia.nih.gov/health/alzheimers/caregiving#pubs.

National Institute on Aging. (2017). Cognitive health and older adults. Retrieved from https://www.nia.nih.gov/health/cognitive-health-and-older-adults#mind.

Pierce, L. (2013). Letting go of resentment and anger as a caregiver. *GoodTherapy.org.* Retrieved from http://www.goodtherapy.org/blog/letting-go-of-resentment-and-anger-as-caregiver-0822135.

Rivera, R. (n.d.). Strategies for coping with caretaker anxiety. *AmericanHomeCare.* Retrieved from http://www.americanhomecare.us/hospice/Strategies%20for%20Coping%20with%20Caretaker%20Anxiety.pdf.

Sauer, A. (2014). 5 reasons why music boosts brain activity. *Alzheimers.net.* Retrieved from https://www.alzheimers.net/why-music-boosts-brain-activity-in-dementia-patients/.

Scott, P. S. (2012). Seven ways to save your relationships from caregiver stress. *Louisiana Weekly.* Retrieved from http://www.louisianaweekly.com/seven-ways-to-save-your-relationships-from-caregiver-stress/.

University of California San Francisco Osher Center for Integrative Medicine. (2018). Guided imagery. Retrieved from https://osher.ucsf.edu/patient-care/treatments/guided-imagery.

University of Michigan: Michigan Medicine. (2018). Stress management: Breathing exercises for relaxation. Retrieved from https://www.uofmhealth.org/health-library/uz2255.

WebMD. (2019). Alzheimer's disease health center. Retrieved from http://www.webmd.com/alzheimers/.

Made in the USA
Middletown, DE
09 February 2023

24422322R00054